72 Ways of Saving Lives

72 WAYS OF SAVING LIVES

FOLK REMEDIES IN OLD CHINA

Ronald Suleski

Foreword by **Shigehisa Kuriyama**

The Chinese University of Hong Kong Press

72 Ways of Saving Lives: Folk Remedies in Old China
 By Ronald Suleski
 Foreword by Shigehisa Kuriyama

© The Chinese University of Hong Kong 2024

ISBN: 978-988-237-321-1

Published by The Chinese University of Hong Kong Press
 The Chinese University of Hong Kong
 Sha Tin, N.T., Hong Kong
 Fax: +852 2603 7355
 Email: cup@cuhk.edu.hk
 Website: cup.cuhk.edu.hk

Printed in Hong Kong

Every effort has been made to trace copyright holders of the illustrations in this book. If any has been inadvertently overlooked, we will be pleased to make the necessary arrangement at the first opportunity.

For my daughters
Kiyomi and Valerie

CONTENTS

FOREWORD

This book offers a translation—with accompanying commentary—of the *Qishier fanzheng*, a nineteenth-century manual of Chinese medicine. But much of the manual's contents will likely be unfamiliar even to specialists of Chinese medical history. We find no mention of the flows and blockages of *qi*, no appeals to the interactions of *yin* and *yang* and the five phases, no concern, in short, with what we have come to imagine as the core elements of Chinese medical thought. What we find, instead, are intriguing puzzles—diseases named after a menagerie of animals, remedies whose logic is often a mystery. And that is what makes this manual so notable and fascinating. It hints at how little we know, even now, about the history of sicknesses and their cures in China.

The seminal works in English that inspired contemporary scholarship on traditional Chinese medicine (TCM) started to appear some forty years ago. The year 1980 saw the publication of *Celestial Lancets* by Lu Gwei-Djen and Joseph Needham, still the major Western-language study of the history of acupuncture. Ted Kaptchuk came out with his influential popularization of Chinese medical thought—*The Web That Has No Weaver*—in 1983, and this was followed in 1985 by the English translation of Paul Unschuld's ambitious survey, *Medicine in China: A History of Ideas*, and in 1987 by Nathan Sivin's translation of a modern TCM textbook, *Traditional Medicine in Contemporary China*.

All of these foundational studies shared one thing in common: they portrayed medicine in China as firmly rooted in major systems of thought—first and foremost in the cosmological theories of *qi*, *yin* and *yang* and the five phases, and secondarily, in the beliefs of Daoism and Buddhism. And this same emphasis on grand philosophical frameworks has continued to characterize most writings about TCM to this day. The motley beliefs and practices falling outside of these intellectual traditions have all been casually lumped together under the label of "folk medicine" and received only occasional, passing mention.

And yet we know that in China, as in the rest of the world, such "folk medicine" was the primary experience of medicine for most people for most of history. Our own ready access to specialists all educated to a shared standard is a historical exception, a recent luxury that is enjoyed, even today, only in some areas of the world. In traditional China, erudite physicians whose diagnoses and therapies were guided by the cosmological reasoning of the *Yellow Emperor's Classic of Medicine* were never more than a tiny elite in a vast sea of diverse healers. Most afflictions were likely handled with the resolute practicality that we find in the *Qishier fanzheng*. It was enough simply to name the disease and apply its remedy. Seeking explanations — asking *why* a disease manifested itself in the way that it did or *why* a particular remedy was supposed to cure it — was superfluous.

Still, today, we cannot help but wonder about these whys. Major parts of the cures proposed in the *Qishier fanzheng* — acupuncture, moxibustion, drugs — are recognizable therapies of TCM. But there are also a good number of less familiar treatments, such as striking parts of the body with shoes or mixing in fluids from masticating horses. And all these elements are deployed in unexpected combinations not found in the classics of acupuncture or the major compendia of pharmacology. A woman is suffering from stomach pains? *Needle the top of her head and the soles of her feet and apply tobacco tar.* A man is shaking his head and wagging his tail? *Needle his forehead and apply the rust of a used hoe three times.* We cannot help but ask: How do acupuncture and tobacco tar work together? Why the rust, specifically, of a used hoe, and why precisely three times? The classical theories of TCM offer little clue. Whatever the latent reasoning behind such treatments, it is clear that folk medicine in China drew on a far more lush and variegated imagination of potencies — a richer sense of the power of diverse places and concrete things — than the bare schemes of *yin-yang* and the five phases.

The specific diseases identified by the *Qishier fanzheng*, too, intimate a vast, unexplored world. There is, to begin, the recurring association of ailments with particular animals — with phoenixes and lambs, mules and horses, snakes, turtles, and toads. What are we to make of this? These associations plainly mattered: the text's illustrations served above all to underscore their primacy. Yet none of the animal names featured in our manual appear in Chao Yuanfang's famous encyclopedia of diseases, the *Zhubing yuanhou lun* (610), and I have yet to find them in later nosological writings. The *Qishier fanzheng*'s evocation of flapping phoenixes and bleating sheep whispers to us of an alternative, radically different approach to diseases of which previous scholarship had given us no intimation.

Nor is it simply the names that are strange. Often, the symptoms with which they are associated are just as puzzling. To be sure, human beings can suffer from a fantastic range of afflictions, and the medical dramas of our own time regularly feature obscure ailments whose manifestations are so bizarre as to verge on the incredible. Outlandish symptoms make for entertaining drama. But *Qishier fanzheng* is, as we have noted, a resolutely practical manual, and compared to the over 1,700 syndromes cataloged in Chao Yuanfang's compendium, 72 represents a very small number. It would seem reasonable to suppose that if the manual's author chose to include a disease in his limited selection it was because the disease was common, because it was a condition whose cure would be necessary in the everyday lives of his readers. And so we are not at all surprised to see prescriptions for such complaints as headaches, stomach pains, and itching. But how often did nineteenth-century Chinese have to deal with patients who flapped their arms like a phoenix? How frequently did one come across sufferers bleating like sheep? And how exactly should we picture the behavior of those afflicted by shaking-head-wagging-tail disease?

The *Qishier fanzheng*, in sum, abounds in engaging enigmas. For much of the four decades scholars have confidently discoursed on Chinese medical thought based on their reading of the *Yellow Emperor's Classic of Medicine* and works composed in its wake. But Professor Suleski's translation and commentary calls our attention to a work that now compels us to expand our horizons—that suggests that the history of Chinese beliefs and practices surrounding sicknesses and their cures may be like the proverbial elephant palpated by blind men: a realm of startling variety and unimaginable immensity of which we have grasped, it turns out, still only a small patch.

Shigehisa Kuriyama
Director, Edwin O. Reischauer Institute of Japanese Studies
Harvard University
February 2024

ACKNOWLEDGEMENTS

As with all efforts in life, this book is the result of help from many friends and specialists. It is my pleasure and honor to thank them here.

Shigehisa "Hisa" Kuriyama 栗山茂久 was gracious in agreeing to write the Foreword. I have admired his lively teaching style at Harvard and am happy he is part of this project. My advisor on medical matters was Li Chen 陳莉 who graduated from the Jiangxi University of Traditional Medicine. Her explanations to me were always well-founded and helpful. Now with a PhD in Marketing, she teaches at the Sawyer Business School at Suffolk University, Boston. It was delightful to find a colleague at my own university who had exactly the expertise I needed for this book project.

My friend in Shanghai, Stone Chen 陳實, teaches at the Shanghai Polytechnic University. He answered many of my questions, and also contacted his medical practitioner friend Gao Yu 高玉 in Shandong, a doctor of traditional Chinese medicine who is accomplished at acupuncture and moxibustion therapy. Dr. Gao conveyed some "on the ground" views of traditional medicine as it is practiced in China today.

Josh Jiaqi Xu 徐嘉啟 did the first transcription into English of the medical recipes while he was a student at Suffolk University. His work was a useful starting point for me. Belal Sohel, then a technology support specialist at Suffolk University, was important to this and other research projects I have carried out and he has scanned in many pages of illustrations for me in the past several years.

At the Harvard-Yenching Library I benefited from the advice and assistance of many friends on the staff. These include: Ma Xiaohe 馬小鶴, Librarian for the Chinese Collection, who has taught me many things over the years about Chinese-language publications; Sharon Li-shiuan Yang 楊麗瑄, the Public Services Librarian, who has been unfailingly friendly and welcoming; and Annie Xi Wang 王繫, Curatorial Assistant for Special Collections, who let me take in my hands the 1916 edition of the *Seventy-Two Therapies* held in their collection.

Equally helpful to me has been the staff at the Sawyer Library at Suffolk, especially the Director Gregory Heald, Manager Sarah Griffis, Senior Reference Librarian Sonia Didriksson, and Becky Shea with Interlibrary Loan Services. Jin Minjie of the Zhejiang Library responded to our request for materials. Huei-Min Jhan 詹惠閔 at the library of the Research Center for Humanities and Social Sciences at the Academia Sinica in Taiwan gave me much information and help in accessing the 1903 edition of the *Seventy-Two Therapies,* and also introduced me to Chu Ping-yi 祝平一 at the Institute of History and Philology at the Academia Sinica, who kindly shared his research and observations about the *Seventy-Two Therapies.* Laura at the Wellcome Collection gave me friendly and useful comments about the 1916 edition put online by the Wellcome Collection in London. Vivienne Lo (Luo Weiqian 羅維前) of University College London also gave me information about the Wellcome online edition and other useful observations on classical Chinese medicine.

Yan Liu 劉焱 at the University at Buffalo, SUNY whose book *Healing with Poisons: Potent Medicines in Medieval China* (Seattle, WA: University of Washington Press, 2021) covered a critical aspect of medical practice in pre-modern China, also gave useful comments on portions of my translated therapies. Barbara Ruth Campbell is a trained medical librarian who located many good sources and forwarded important medical observations to me in regard to many of the medical recipes I was working on. Jonghyun Lee gave me a number of crucial insights and suggestions for this project. I am grateful for his continued support for my research.

I benefitted greatly from the expertise, insights, and friendliness of the editorial team at The Chinese University of Hong Kong Press. They included: Ye Minlei 葉敏磊, Senior Acquisitions Editor and Editorial Manager, who always encouraged me in this project; Brian M. C. Yu 余敏聰, Editor, who impressed me with his thoroughness, his knowledge of all aspects of processing the manuscript into a printed book, and his quick responses to every one of my enquiries; and Angelina Lai-fun Wong 黃麗芬, then Business Manager, who actually remembered working on my earlier publication with the Press in 1994—I am sure both of us smiled at that nice connection.

A generous grant from the Rosenberg Institute for East Asian Studies at Suffolk University, Boston was approved by the RI Advisory Council toward the publication of this book. I take responsibility for all errors in this study.

Ronald Suleski
April 2024

Introduction and Interpretive Overview

The Seventy-Two Medical Therapies

How did lay people in old China save their lives when dealing with acute or chronic health issues? Conventional medicine was costly and might not have been an option for many. Instead, people in villages and towns relied on remedies drawn from a woodblock-printed illustrated booklet called *Seventy-Two Therapies* (*Qishier fanzheng* 七十二翻症), first published in 1847.

Among the recommended remedies, the ashes of a grasshopper (*jila* 蟣蠟) could relieve muscle cramps, while powdered mulberry leaves (*sangye* 桑葉) would reduce swelling of the limbs. These were among the traditional ingredients and treatment methods readily available to the common people wherever they lived.

Depending on the health issues present, sometimes they drank an herbal powder mixed in yellow rice wine. At other times the recommendation was to apply acupuncture, the mud from a hornet's nest, or a bit of cat urine, combined with a slap to shock their system out of erratic behavior. The remedy would work fairly quickly to relieve the worst of the symptoms within the same day. Each page of the *Seventy-Two Therapies* is the product of China's recorded folk wisdom. Happily, contemporary scientific analysis shows that the traditional Chinese approaches to relieving distress also bring relief for modern maladies such as respiratory symptoms, the side effects of chemotherapy, or even inhibiting the growth of tumors. The goal of this book is to foster an appreciation of China's long tradition of folk remedies.[1] It is a tradition that belongs to all humankind.

This manual of medical problems and quick treatments was circulating in China in the 1860s. Today, it has become almost a lost treasure of China's tradition of folk remedies. It is not listed in many of the medical dictionaries published in China! Yet since its first appearance in the mid-1800s, it has been pirated and reprinted many times, and it can be found in a printed version and an online edition today. What a fate to befall a text that has been a friend to the Chinese people for so many years. It was intended to be an inexpensive and convenient guide offering immediate relief to people suffering from a malady that was bringing them discomfort. It was also intended as a quick reference for people in need of emergency medical attention. There can be no question that a lot of people have consulted this manual.

The manual is a collection of accepted folk remedies that emerged from China's long tradition of medical research. Searching online I found a paragraph describing this work. My translation/adaptation of that paragraph reads: "The *Seventy-Two Therapies* is a classic document of how Chinese traditional medicine (*Zhongyi* 中醫) provides emergency medical treatment for various syndromes. Its illustrations and graphics are as simple as can be, but the medical theories behind the prescriptions are well-founded. Chinese traditional medicine holds that every disease has a specific pathology. The internal organs are sensitive, exposed to pathogens, and have correspondences with other aspects of the living body. Finding those points and dealing with them in a timely and effective manner can instantly save people's lives. Some of the prescribed therapies sound cruel, such as the hot needle therapy (*huozhen liaofa* 火針療法) or large needle therapies (*juzhen liaofa* 巨針療法). But they are actually unique life-saving skills. We can only guess at how many lives have been saved since ancient times by using these techniques. This approach is definitely worth our attention."[2]

The size of the woodblock copy I bought at the Panjiayuan Antiques Market (*Panjiayuan jiuhuo shichang* 潘家園舊貨市場) in Beijing in June 2013 is small, just 6 inches (15.24 cm) tall and 4.5 inches (11.43 cm) wide. It is a perfect size to fit into a pocket of the kind of short jacket (*magua* 馬褂) widely worn in the Qing Dynasty (1644–1911). The handmade paper, now matured to a light brown color because of the bamboo and rice stalks used in its manufacture, is very pliable and lightweight. Each page gives a brief explanation of the presenting symptoms of the patient, and then suggests a medical treatment. The medicine usually prescribed calls for a few herbs to be burnt into a fine powder (*shaohuang wei mo* 燒黃為末). Often the powder was put into the mouth and swallowed down with a cup of tea or yellow rice wine (*huangjiu* 黃酒). It was also common to dissolve the powdered herbs in the liquid and have the patient drink the warmed liquid.[3]

For most people in China throughout history, the logic of illness was straightforward. Feeling ill, then take some medicine. Prepare the medicine and drink it. That was the approach then and now, and it constitutes the basis of how people think of the traditional Chinese reaction to illness, using herbs and naturally occurring ingredients as much as possible. The medicine was often prepared in the home.[4]

Each page of the manual translated here has a few points of the presenting symptoms (*qi xing* 其形), and the basic recipe for preparing the medicine. Each page also has a simplified line drawing of a typical patient in distress because of their symptoms. By convention, the medical conditions in the booklet were associated with an animal or living creature, such as a cicada (*qiuchan* 秋蟬), chicken (*ji* 雞), lizard (*xiehu* 蠍虎), or horse (*ma* 馬), and the identifying animal was also drawn on each page as a quick reference. It could be that the patient was acting like the animal shown in the drawing, or only because the name of the animal drawn was adopted over the centuries as a way to label the disease.

Linking these illness behaviors to some animal or insect was actually a clever and very useful device. Throughout the hundreds of years of medical research in China, thousands of medical recipes had been developed. Most were listed in terms of the ingredients they used. While the highly trained medical scholar or pharmacist had knowledge about many of them, the typical rural medical practitioner in all likelihood did not. Especially in an emergency situation when being confronted by a person in need of medical attention, a quick response was called for. The brief designation of each problem would provide the most rapid way to locate a potentially useful remedy. A semi-literate person could find the drawings useful to quickly find the information they were seeking.

The reasoning behind the name (label) assigned to each therapy is not always clear. For example, the patient might act as if they were some creature from the animal world, crawling along the ground or loudly baying, and so the patient's affliction would be given the name of an animal which acted in that manner. Or the patient would feel as if some insects were crawling on their body, leading to the name of that insect being given to the affliction. I conclude this logic of naming was a type of "sympathetic naming," in the sense of linking the insect- or animal-produced expression of the affliction and thus symbolically connecting those creatures to the disease and its cure. One could also say the labels on each therapy reflect a folk quality of the medicine, that it was basic medicine often prescribed for and self-administered by the common people (*pingmin* 平民). The animals and insects that provided the names of most of the illnesses listed were all common to a rural population including, especially for those in north China around Beijing, the camel (the remedy discussed in P25) that was until recent times widely used to transport goods.[5]

When a person in old China expressed physical discomfort, even a severe headache or a painful stomach, or when someone was seen to be acting in an unnatural manner, such as being very unsteady on their feet, it was clear to their relatives and others around them that a medical problem was manifesting itself and some remedy was called for. The natural inclination was to turn to the family members of the distressed person. In many cases we expect the first reaction of potential caregivers was to ask family members to suggest a therapy. Perhaps a grandparent could suggest a broth to take away the pain, or an uncle might have seen the condition before and knew of a remedy. In other words, the first response was usually to try to devise a way of receiving help without incurring any special expense; not many people had surplus cash laying around the house for medicine. It was likely felt best to avoid calling on a doctor, pharmacist, or a literate person who practiced giving medical advice, because there would be some expense incurred, whether the payment of money or a suitable "thank you" gift for help received.

There was no national system in China for training or certifying medical practitioners in the Qing Dynasty which ended in 1911. The Chinese Medical Association (*Zhonghua yixuehui* 中華醫學會), the largest and oldest non-governmental medical organization in China, was established under the Republic in 1915 based on the influences of Western medical associations. The idea was to standardize and evaluate the medical training students received and to follow the latest medical thinking of doctors in Western countries. They had the influence of the Western medical missionaries who were working in China during the Qing period and practiced Western-style medicine. In the political dislocations that followed in China between 1915 and 1950, medical education and certifications never achieved a single standard that was followed throughout the country.

In the late 1800s when the manual translated here began to be printed and circulated, there was not the concept of medical doctors being highly specialized. Offering medical advice or remedies was a private business taken up by some people. Up to that time literate people, those who had at least a few years of formal schooling and who could read and write, often included medicine among the subjects they encountered in their studies. When faced with someone in trouble, the first non-family person turned to for help was one of the literate people in the vicinity. Whether a family relative or a nearby literate person, the knowledge base from which they drew information was the tradition of Chinese folk remedies.

We can picture the person who was practicing as a medical doctor and was called on to visit a patient in distress. The patient was perhaps beset by purple-red blotches (*ding* 疔) on their body or was acting in a strange manner, maybe rolling on the ground or curled in a fetal position. Those were the emergency situations when the doctor or informal medical practitioner needed to quickly offer some relief. From the symptoms the practitioner noted, a treatment could be given. The prescriptions offered on each page of this manual are not especially complicated and the herbal ingredients would have been available at most pharmacies (*yaoju* 藥局) in China in those times.[6] In fact, all of the remedies explained in this booklet called for herbs and items that were likely to be available in every city or village, even when a pharmacy was not nearby. We can see that there was a preference in the recommended therapies for ingredients that would easily be found in the rural farming villages.

China's Tradition of Medical Research:
The *Yellow Emperor's Classic of Medicine*

The description above of what was taking place in the 1860s and the role of the manual in providing guidance appears simple and straightforward. In the old China prior to 1950, formally trained medical doctors were few. Many people logically assumed that a person who was literate, someone who could read and write, had knowledge beyond that of the typical person who could not read or write well and who had limited formal education. People in the cities or villages often knew of someone who, because of their literacy, could tell fortunes, or advise on the proper way to conduct weddings or funerals, or to treat a person in physical distress. When some sort of medical intervention was called for, and after the immediate family decided they were unable to help, they would contact the nearest literate person known to them. As mentioned above, it might be a relative or an older person living nearby who already had a reputation for giving useful medical advice.

In spite of the widespread use of accepted "folk remedies" based on stories handed down by the common people, China had a tradition of literate persons who actively examined substances for their medical properties. They would test the effectiveness of these herbs or substances when they could, compare their effects, then list and categorize them. In addition, there were theories about how the body functioned, why disease occurred, how to explain the effectiveness of particular herbs and decoctions in the process of curing the body. Thus developed an orderly and detailed corpus of knowledge about the bodily processes of living things, the effects and side effects of accepted treatments, and written records of these findings.[7]

The people living in a city or village who were able to call upon someone who knew about this tradition of medical thinking and research were fortunate, because they had found a person who was aware of the long history of medical thinking in China. The classic work explaining the basis for medical thinking and analysis was and still is the *Yellow Emperor's Classic of Medicine* (*Huangdi neijing* 黃帝內經). It introduces the theoretical foundation of Chinese Medicine and its diagnostic methods. The thinking of this text is based on an analytical structure about the origin of the world and the actions of the forces within it that was well-established by the time it was compiled, likely before the end of the Han Dynasty (206 BCE–220 CE). The *Yellow Emperor's Classic* took that analytical structure as the basis for explaining the functioning of the human body. For example, the universe of all phenomena, the myriad things (*wanwu* 萬物), contained a vital force called *qi* 氣 that propelled the elements into motion. Each element within the universe contained degrees of dark, cool, negative (*yin* 陰) forces, or bright, hot, positive (*yang* 陽) forces. These two qualities of *yin-yang* interacted with each other seeking a balance, or harmony, or an accommodation allowing each to co-exist.[8]

Of these critical aspects of life, the concept of the vital force of *qi* is the most difficult to translate and define in English. The scholar Vivienne Lo has provided a succinct discussion of *qi* by writing: "*Qi* (sometimes rendered *ch'i*) is a complex and changing concept which defies simple lineal histories. In the mid–Warring States, references to it tend to refer to atmospheric and environmental conditions, especially moist vapours — clouds and mists — and, by analogy, to formless, clustering qualities that can be discerned with careful observation, like smoke, ghosts or the vibrant, martial aura of an army. By the mid-4th century *qi* often indicates the fundamental stuff in nature which both promotes and indicates vitality in the phenomenal world. It may enter the body in various ways — through the orifices and the skin — but its movement within the body is not formalized. Some historians translate *qi* as 'vapour' and, in doing so, underline the amorphous watery qualities of steam and mist, which are formative influences both in the early period and as an enduring feature of the concept. As *qi* begins to be applied to the phenomena of the inner body, the ideas, although never totally distinct from the early versions, go through significant transformations. Rather than replacing the old meanings, the range of meanings grows incrementally — a process that is continuous to the present day."[9]

Just as this elemental conjunction of all the forces outlined above could explain the change of the seasons, the effects of natural processes, and the influence of the stars on human beings, it could also be used to explain how the human body worked. Aspects of the natural world affected the health and vigor of the human body. For example, critical to the continuation of human life is blood (*xue* 血), which flows throughout the body by the force of *qi*. Multiple factors internal or external to the body will affect how smoothly the blood flows or is prevented from flowing. Organs of the body might be invaded by dry heat (*zaore* 燥熱) causing fever, excitability, or skin rash. The pathogen (*xie* 邪; the word means evil spirit) could be a malicious wind (*efeng* 惡風) or a damp cold (*shihan* 濕寒), causing vomiting, chills, or listlessness. [10]

The Yellow Emperor is considered to be a culture hero, a mythical ruler who appeared at the beginning of the formation of the Chinese cultural complex. But the ideas and their interactions that emerged from the *Yellow Emperor's Classic* in a form more elaborate and complicated than outlined here, became the basis for medical thinking that still forms the worldview of what today is widely known as Traditional Chinese Medicine (TCM).[11]

Current Western thinking is that the TCM movement was an effort by the government of the People's Republic to buttress Chinese traditional medical practices, after they were praised by Mao Zedong in the 1950s, into an aspect of Chinese culture that could gain worldwide respect and would come to be seen as an equal to the widely respected practices of Western medical

research. This is in fact happening in the world today. Some Western scholars think the Chinese medical tradition represents a huge body of historical
research, classification, and analysis, and should not be codified and "isolated"
from human medical knowledge. Instead, they think that the scientific rigor
of the Western method needs to be applied to the Chinese medical tradition
and the claims of Chinese doctors need to be verified according to strict scientific analysis.[12] This is also happening in the world today, as my comments on
the remedies translated in this book illustrate.

China's Tradition of Medical Research: Early Researchers

Hua Tuo

By the time the Han Dynasty ended in 220 CE, China was well into its historical period, when many written records were available. Scholars who
studied the cosmological principles of the time experimented with medical
treatments. They were to become the first medical specialists in China and
prepared written records of their work. Well-known among them is Hua Tuo
華佗, believed to have lived circa 145–208 CE in the late Eastern Han Dynasty.
Historical records describing those days such as the *Records of the Three Kingdoms* (*Sanguozhi* 三國志) and *Book of the Later Han* (*Houhanshu* 後漢書) talk
about his medical work. Some scholars believe he learned Ayurveda medical
techniques from the early Indian Buddhist missionaries in China. Ayurveda
thinking emphasizes good health and the prevention and treatment of illness
through following a healthy lifestyle while practicing massage, meditation,
and yoga, along with nourishing foods and the use of herbal remedies. It is a
wholistic approach that pulls together the effects of both the natural and the
physical world to create an environment to sustain good health in the human
body.[13]

Hua Tuo practiced surgery, cutting open the human body as a way to
understand the origin of the physical discomfort and to restore smooth bodily
functioning. He is credited with being the first person in China to use anes-
thesia during surgery. His general anesthetic combined wine with a herbal
decoction called boiled hemp powder (*mafeisan* 麻沸散). The word *ma* 麻 indicates an herb that served as a numbing agent and the term *dama* 大麻 is used
to refer to cannabis or marijuana. He also used early forms of acupuncture,
moxibustion, and the role of physical exercise in aiding good health.

Hua Tuo observed the movement of animals and from his observations is credited with the development of a set of exercises designed to strengthen human muscles. These are called the Exercise of the Five Animals (*Wuqinxi* 五禽戲) and have been adopted by some schools of Chinese martial arts as part of their training regimen. Taking traditional information and applying it to the present day is part of the Chinese practice in all areas of maintaining good health. An important point in terms of the *Seventy-Two Therapies* is that Hua Tuo's broad approach established the connection between considering illnesses and their cures by referring to animals and other sentient organisms, a connection which is illustrated on almost every page of the manual translated here, since sentient creatures are represented so frequently as a quick reference to the remedy outlined on the page. For his work in understanding the internal organs of the human body, Hua Tuo is honored as the Divine Physician (*Shenyi* 神醫).[14]

Zhang Zhongjing

Another early highly respected medical researcher was Zhang Zhongjing 張仲景 (Zhongjing is his courtesy name [*zi* 字] and he is sometimes listed by his given name as Zhang Ji 張機), whose approximate dates are 150–219 CE. His major contribution to Chinese medical knowledge was his work as a pharmacologist. He collected and studied plants that could be "purified" through grinding and boiling, and so put to use for their medical properties. He studied as many medicinal plants and herbs as he could find, identifying the internal organs they could affect and the types of medical conditions for which they could be applied. Although his written materials were lost, succeeding scholars have reconstructed much of his work.

One of his areas of research was on the damage caused by cold pathogens (*hanxie* 寒邪) that brought on many of the epidemic infectious diseases resulting in fevers that were prevalent during the era in which he lived. His lost research was collected in the book *Treatise of Cold Pathogenic and Miscellaneous Diseases* (*Shanghan zabing lun* 傷寒雜病論). Linking adverse medical conditions to extreme heat or cold is one of the hallmarks of the traditional Chinese approach to understanding the causes of physical discomfort and it is a basis on which these age-old analytical categories are practiced in China, Korea, Japan, and Vietnam.[15]

Cold (*han* 寒) can affect the body, not only by low temperatures, but by a wind (*feng* 風) or a dampness (*shi* 濕) that enters the body to lodge in the inner organs. Thus, a person even in a warm climate can become ill when this happens. Zhang Zhongjing's ideas fostered a school of thought among Chinese doctors of regularly seeking the location of the cold pathogen within the body, and determining which herbal decoctions could be used to dislodge the heat and to restore smooth functioning to the body. Many of the therapies in this manual refer to the presence of wind or dampness. Removing the debilitating heat would remove the imbalances in the patient. Japanese doctors refer to this school of thought as the Theory of Fevers (*netsu ron* 熱論).[16]

The thrust of Zhang's research dealt with the damage caused by cold (*shanghan* 傷寒) and was a study of febrile diseases, which are illnesses that cause a fever. As most of us know, a fever is often the first thing we check for when a person complains of feeling unwell. Today Zhang Zhongjing is honored as the Sage of Chinese Medicine (*Yisheng* 醫聖).

Sun Simiao

The most prominent of these early physicians and the one best known to the Chinese people today was Sun Simiao 孫思邈. He lived during the Sui and Tang Dynasties (581–907 CE) and is said to have died in 682. He was a prolific scholar who made many contributions to understanding the applications of medical thinking to treating patients. In his work *Essential Formulas Worth a Thousand Cash to Prepare for Emergencies* (*Beiji qianjin yaofang* 備急千金要方) he listed over 5,300 recipes for medicines, and in a supplementary work *Medical Formulas Worth a Thousand Cash* (*Qianjin yaofang* 千金要方) he added 2,000 more medical recipes. Note that the phrase "A Thousand Cash" (*qianjin* 千金) carries the meaning of being essential or invaluable. It is a phrase taken from the everyday language of the common people of his day and has continued to be used into modern times.

Sun Simiao's work covered many of the areas still of importance in Chinese traditional medicine as it is practiced today and that constitute the categories of basic knowledge that a Chinese practitioner should know. Among these are antidotes and detoxification (*jiedu jijiu* 解毒急救), pulse diagnostics (*maixue* 脈學), acupuncture and moxibustion (*zhenjiu* 針灸), massage (*tuina* 推拿), bonesetting (*dieda* 跌打), and others. Sun concentrated on how internal medicine operates in relation to coldness and heat, in particular to deficiency (*xu* 虛) and excess (*shi* 實) in the internal organs (viscera, *zangfu* 臟腑). He also wrote about women's illnesses (gynecology) and the diseases of children (pediatrics). All of these topics are covered in the manual translated here.[17]

Sun Simiao is venerated as the King of Medicine (*Yaowang* 藥王). Many statues of him were carved in the past two hundred years and were placed on the altars of Daoist temples or in family homes. Many of these figures of the King of Medicine taken from old temples are for sale in the antiques stores of Liulichang 琉璃廠 in Beijing today.[18] It seems to me that when I say the name of Sun Simiao in China, everyone immediately recognizes the name, which they confirm by linking him to medicine and health.

All three of these early medical practitioners—Hua Tuo, Zhang Zhongjing, and Sun Simiao—are honored as Daoist deities in the Medicine King Hall (*Yaowangdian* 藥王殿) of the White Cloud Monastery (*Baiyunguan* 白雲觀) in Beijing. These three worthies have been grouped by Daoist thinking as the preeminent researchers who helped to form the core of practical and applied knowledge in the long tradition of Chinese folk remedies. Persons who ask for good health for themselves, their grandparents, parents and children come to this Hall, often visibly upset and emotional, offering foods and flowers, and burning incense outside the Hall to ask for their help. The Hall, one of the busiest in this monastery complex, receives a steady stream of visitors of all ages bowing, kneeling, and offering prayers. I have been among them.[19] A wood carving of Sun Simiao originally at a Daoist temple rests on my desk (see Appendix B) as I write this in Cambridge, Massachusetts.

We should keep in mind that the preeminent figures in China's medical research such as those mentioned here, relied on many students and fellow investigators to carry out the studies and experiments that led to the present-day definitions and uses of the remedies and medical practices in China's long history of medical research. These studies were carried out over many years and often in widely separated locations. Sometimes the teacher worked with a small group of students, and at other times individual researchers gathered their information and analysis, then sent the information on to their teacher. Because of the constant exchange of information among the investigators, the conclusions reached, both in terms of theoretical insights and applied medicine, should be respected as the results of team efforts based on many years of study.

China's Tradition of Medical Research: Classifying Herbs

Li Shizhen

Most of the remedies presented in this translated manual prescribe plants and herbs that can be used to alleviate the problems besetting a patient. These constitute the most practical application of Chinese traditional folk remedies, and are a characteristic of the traditional approach to dealing with medical issues. This medical approach is the most widely practiced throughout East Asia. For example, when the Japanese speak of "Chinese Medicine" (*kanpōyaku* 漢方藥), as is widely advertised in Japan today, the medicine (*yaku* 藥) to which they refer are medicinal plants and herbs.

A notable corpus of work on the use of medical analysis and the use of herbs to compound medical recipes is the amazing *Compendium of Materia Medica* (*Bencao gangmu* 本草綱目). Earlier records about medicinal herbs were combined, carefully classified and updated in this second classical book related to the *Yellow Emperor's Classic* universally used by doctors in China and throughout East Asia where this traditional style of medicine is practiced. The *Materia Medica* is a multi-volume work; its first draft was completed in 1578 and it was published and printed from woodblocks in Nanjing, China in 1596. It has stood the test of time for accuracy and completeness and is the basis for much of the information on the therapeutic use of plants and herbs in Chinese folk remedies. The medical researcher Li Shizhen 李時珍 (1518–1593) spent nearly thirty years collecting, analyzing, classifying, and commenting on as many medicinal plants as he could acquire.

The table of contents contains a list of entries included and has 1,160 hand-drawn diagrams to serve as illustrations. It has an index (*xuli* 序例) and an extensive list of herbs that can be used to treat the most common sickness (*baibing zhuzhiyao* 百病主治藥). The main body of the text contains 1,892 specific herbs, and it is said that 374 of these were added by Li Shizhen himself. There are 11,096 additional prescriptions to treat the most common illnesses, of which 8,160 are compiled in the text. For every herb there are entries on their names, with a detailed description of their appearance and smell, their nature, medical functions, noted side effects, and how they can be used in medical recipes. It is truly a comprehensive work.[20]

The 1500s was a time when Western thinkers and researchers in Europe were also forming theories and methodically working through medical problems. Was there contact between the Chinese researchers in Asia and the Persian and European researchers in the West? By the time of Li Shizhen's extensive compilation, there had already been well over a thousand years of contact between both Eastern and Western civilizations over the Silk Road (*Sichou zhi lu* 絲綢之路), which was in full operation by 100 BCE. But we need to keep in mind that the world of the 1500s was vast because travel took so very long. Further, much of the world was unknown to the great majority of people living in the other civilizations. We might suppose that contacts between Asia, Persia, and the West were speeded up and increased in number during the Great Mongol Empire of 1206–1368, when the Mongol armies of Genghis Khan ruled a territory stretching from Korea in the east to European Russia and Poland in the west. In comparison to earlier times, the movement of people, books, and knowledge was greatly facilitated by the relatively unified administrative systems set in place under the Mongols. The administrative systems were not overly complicated and were quite tolerant of the people and goods moving among the administrative centers. As a result, people, goods, languages, and ideas flowed freely over the thousands of miles of the "known" world.[21]

The 1860s manual translated here is filled with information based very closely on the classifications and medical prescriptions expounded in this *Compendium of Materia Medica* that had appeared in China some 260 years earlier. The thinking among the peoples of East Asia about the importance of herbal medicine was widespread. In neighboring Korea, where traditional Chinese folk remedies was called "Chinese medicine" (*hanyak* 한약, 漢藥), not only the common people but the highest elites as well were treated with herbal decoctions. Traditional Chinese folk remedies were respected throughout Korean society and were the first medical interventions turned to when a patient was in distress.[22]

Chinese traditional folk remedies also influenced medical practices in Vietnam. The Vietnamese tended to less frequently use the medical decoctions prescribed by the Chinese tradition, and as might be expected, they used herbs and plants more common to their own climate. Those plants included herbs and vegetables such as laksa leaves (*rau răm, leshaye* 叻沙葉), marjoram (*la kinh giới, mayulan* 馬郁蘭), chrysanthemum (*cải cúc, juhua* 菊花), spinach (*rau muống, bocai* 菠菜), or flowers such as *Magnolia champaca* (*yulan* 玉蘭), a large evergreen tree of the magnolia family, and *Jasminum sambac* (*shaba moli* 沙巴

茉莉), a species of jasmine native to tropical Asia. The plants tended to be used in their fresh state or simply dried. Occasionally, animal products such as silkworms would be prescribed. Traditional medical prescriptions could be applied through ingested preparations, ointments, and the poultice. A poultice is a hot, soft mass of a paste or plants, often wrapped in a damp cloth, that is placed on the body to relieve soreness and inflammation.[23]

A Word on Acupuncture

Running parallel to the great interest in using herbs and plants for medical treatment was the use of acupuncture (*zhenjiu* 針灸).[24] This term referred both to the use of needles and the practice of moxibustion, applying heat to affected areas of the body. Regarding needles, this was the use of needles inserted into the skin of the patient in order to clear blockages in the flow of blood throughout the system. Blood flowed through the meridians (*jingmai* 經脈) or channels (*jingluo* 經絡) and any interruption to the flow negatively impacted the internal organs linked to the meridians, causing illnesses.[25] Sometimes the lack of smooth blood flow caused a physical reaction that was visible to the attending physician. A common reaction seen throughout the manual translated here were the pustules (*ding* 疔) mentioned above, discolored raised portions on the skin filled with pus or red-purple-black eruptions caused by accumulations of blood, similar to pimples. This could be accompanied by a swelling of the skin, or a rash, or a discoloration on parts of the body. The ideas about meridians and channels, and the eruption of pustules all related to the theories behind acupuncture.[26]

Even the earliest researchers such as Hua Tuo experimented with pricking the skin to help relieve pain and restore health to the body.[27] In traditional medicine the needles were used in combination with other treatments, usually with a prepared medicinal powder made from herbs and drunk with tea or wine. In current practice with the popularity of acupuncture today in both Asia and the West, the needles are used to relieve aches and pains and are often part of a larger prescribed regimen of healthy eating and exercise. These days acupuncture can be prescribed to alleviate simple aches and pains, soreness or even headaches brought on by stress.

Acupuncture became more popular among the Chinese people from the 1800s on. As mentioned above, after 1950 the communist government of the

People's Republic of China promoted the use of acupuncture as part of the scientific heritage of Chinese culture. They began use of the term Traditional Chinese Medicine (TCM) to refer to the body of medical thinking, including acupuncture, herbal medicines, and other medical techniques that had been created by Chinese scholars over the centuries. It was their way to honor traditional Chinese folk wisdom and the huge body of medical research it reflected.

The materials deemed best suited for acupuncture and the exact measurements of needles were publicized by medical researchers from the 1950s on with the approval of the Chinese government. Modern technology allows very thin and sturdy needles to be manufactured to replace the earlier needles of a thicker diameter. It seems that earlier needles were not standardized: some could be rather thick, and they might not always be sharp. Modern needles are precisely made, usually very thin, yet sturdy and can be sterilized. In modern times while using better needles, Chinese doctors carried forward research to determine the exact location of acupuncture points on the human body, so the placement of the needles on the body became more exact and standardized.[28]

Many acupuncture points had been identified in earlier times and most had a poetically descriptive name based on traditional thinking about how the meridians worked inside the body. Among the poetic names are: Union Valley (*hegu* 合谷, classified as LI-4), located on the hand in the fleshy area between the thumb and index finger; it looks like a valley when the hand is relaxed. Celestial Pivot (*tianshu* 天樞, classified as ST-25), located just below the navel; it is near the belly button which is the central point of the human body. Gate of the Soul (*hunmen* 魂門, classified as BL-47), located near the 9th thoracic vertebra on the spinal column; the *hun* is the spiritual soul which can leave the body after death.

At present there are twelve major meridians, and some lists claim over 2,000 acupuncture points. Since the 1950s acupuncture points have also been given letter and number designations, as seen above. To use as an example an acupuncture point mentioned in this manual in P2, when the arm is bent there is a crease that forms toward the side (lateral) of the arm. At the end of this crease is the acupuncture point labeled Pool at the Bend (*quchi* 曲池).[29] It is on the meridian that links to the large intestine (*dachangjing* 大腸經). The letter-number classification of this meridian is LI (large intestine). It starts from the tip of the index finger at acupuncture point NI-1, and continues to point LI-20 near the nostril of the nose. The Pool at the Bend is classified as acupuncture point LI-11. Along this route the internal meridian connects with the stomach channel (*weijing* 胃經) at the acupuncture point labeled ST-25 (ST means stomach) at the Celestial Pivot (*tianshu* 天樞) mentioned above, where the effects of its movement enter the large intestine.

An interesting case of a sensitive area not lying on a meridian but co-opted as a special acupuncture point is the area between the two eyebrows. This is a pressure point (discussed in P38 in this manual) where it is not uncommon when we feel tired or have a headache to put pressure from our thumb and forefinger at this place on our forehead. We have all seen people pinch the area of the upper nose between the eyes when worried or feeling exhaustion. It is called the Hall of Impressions (*yintang* 印堂, sometimes in English the "third eye"), and can be used to treat anxiety, frontal headache, and nasal obstruction. It is considered a non-channel acupuncture point because it does not lie on a meridian.[30]

In the case explained in P2 in this manual, the doctor selected the LI meridian because that seemed to be the particular channel that was not functioning properly based on the presenting symptoms of the patient. Ultimately the large intestine would be involved, but the immediate point to be stimulated or corrected was on the LI meridian. In the manual translated here, based on the medical approach of the 1860s, very few acupuncture points are mentioned. The manual illustrates the interaction between both acupuncture and herbal decoctions to bring relief from the patient's medical complaint and both approaches appear in the remedies listed in the manual.

Chinese Medical Practice in the 1860s

Such were the intellectual foundations that the Chinese practitioner in the 1860s called upon when confronted with a person in need of medical attention. In those days the majority of people in China had very few years of formal schooling. Most lived in rural areas and engaged in manual labor. Although many people could probably read and write a few characters, most were unable to write a letter or to read a book. Those who had received three, five, or more years of formal education were looked up to as literate and knowledgeable. They might have passed the county or prefectural examination and had the status of student (*shengyuan* 生員) or were awarded the title of flourishing talent (*xiucai* 秀才). In the view of most people, those with formal education were knowledgeable about many things because they had read widely and had a broader view of all subject matter. An educated person could be a teacher, a fortuneteller, an advisor on legal matters, a ritual specialist who read from texts, a master of calligraphy, and so forth. People who had received even this "basic" degree received general respect from ordinary people.

Many of the people who could read and write worked a little bit in several of these literate professions at the same time. Among the typical work to be followed by an educated person was that of a medical doctor. In my translations of this manual, I sometimes refer to them as doctors, herbal doctors, or practitioners. Their level of formal education was not always high, but no doubt a good number of them had gained much practical experience over the years and came to be respected as effective healers.[31]

Books about medical information were also widely available in China in the 1860s. People have always been interested in matters of health and sickness, and the use of woodblocks allowed texts to be illustrated and for hundreds of copies to be produced from a single woodblock set. Later in the 1890s lithography (*shiyin* 石印) came to China and was in general use by publishers. This system allowed woodblock editions, both text and illustrations, to be inexpensively copied from an image and printed. Versions of the *Seventy-Two Therapies* were also printed in lithograph copies. Several of the copies of the *Seventy-Two Therapies* currently available on the internet are lithograph editions, but the manual in my collection is a woodblock-printed edition. It has been suggested that copies of this work were sometimes distributed *gratis*, either as a way of wishing good health for those receiving the manual, or as a "promotional" text to draw in paying patients.[32]

Many of the people who practiced medicine treated their medical knowledge as a secret, something they would pass along to their students but otherwise would preserve for themselves as part of their own privileged information. They preserved their knowledge by keeping the medical information only in hand-written versions (*shouxieben* 手寫本). In China, one can find many copies of hand-written medical texts for sale in the antiques markets, along with ledgers of medical recipes about the herbs and preparations for specific therapies. In my collection of medical texts, many are hand-written.[33] But there were a lot of people who did not have the money to acquire any substantial amount of medical information, nor the education to allow them to copy out medical texts. For those people at the lower end of the economic scale, the thin woodblock edition of the manual translated here was as if a gift from the gods. Everything was simplified to its most basic elements. The presenting symptoms of the patient were listed in a few brief remarks. Something about the patient's demeanor or actions were indicated in the line illustration on the page. Many of the individual therapies had by custom been given a label, usually referring to an animal or insect, which made it an easier way to remember the different medical conditions and the treatment prescribed. If the doctors themselves could not read all of the characters on the page, they could find someone who would read them aloud, and the medical practitioner would easily understand what was written.

My Copy of the *Seventy-Two Therapies*

The medical manual that I bought in Beijing that June day in 2013 had lost its original cover, so its exact title and information about its printing or compiler or date of printing were lost to me. Someone had replaced the original front and back covers on my copy with sheets of inexpensive handmade paper and had written on the cover *Ways to Cure Illness* (*Bingzhifang* 病治方). That is a clear descriptive title but may not have been the original title of the book.

As stated above in this Introduction, the manual translated here is a version of a standard collection of medical information known as the *Seventy-Two Therapies* (*Qishier fanzheng* 七十二翻症). It might also be translated as *Curing the Seventy-Two Diseases*. A number of versions of this collection were produced and were for sale in China through the late Qing and Republican periods up to 1950. After the People's Republic was established in 1949, the lithographed copies were reprinted several times in the 1950s. A renewed interest in the folk remedies in the manual arose in the 1970s and 1990s. I have found multiple versions of these editions available on the internet, on sites from mainland China, Taiwan, England, and a Korean bookseller with a Chinese version of this for sale in 2019.[34] I used the copies of these manuals available online as a way to evaluate and compare them to the copy in my collection.

Chinese researchers have historically liked to classify categories by assigning them a number. For instance, in 1973 a medical text was discovered in the Mawangdui 馬王堆 tomb in Changsha, China that had been sealed in 168 BCE. Its title was *Recipes for Fifty-Two Ailments* (*Wushier bingfang* 五十二病方). It contains more than 250 exorcistic and drug-based cures for ailments such as warts, hemorrhoids, and snake bites. So the manual *Seventy-Two Therapies* in my collection was titled based on a tradition of numbering like things into distinct categories, a practice that is well-established among the Chinese.

There are versions of this title on the internet that indeed contain seventy-two recipes, but the copy in my collection contains eighty-one recipes. Each of these is illustrated, except for the final twenty-one which are text-only; they do not have an illustration of either a patient in distress or a related animal caricature. Moreover, in my copy eleven pages are missing, meaning twenty-two additional recipes which might have been in the booklet are not there.

It appears the collection of seventy-two medical recipes contained the most widely used folk remedies. From what I have seen, different editions of this set of medical prescriptions did not all contain the same prescriptions. It seems likely that some of the prescriptions usually seen in this set of *Seventy-Two Therapies* were on the pages that had been removed from my copy. Versions of the *Seventy-Two Therapies* reprinted in the early 1900s had remedies that were not in my collection, and we know that a set of the seventy-two could contain more than that number. Suffice it to say that this was not a fixed collection of therapies. I think we can safely say, however, that because of the many times they were reprinted, the basic medical recipes in these collections were the most popular prescriptions made by doctors and followed by the common people of China.

Why were various pages missing from my woodblock copy? One possible explanation is that at some point the string binding was removed and the set was rebound with a new string. Some of the pages may have "fallen out" at that point and were not rebound. I prefer another explanation. In my copy, for example, folio page 16, composed of sides "a" and "b," has had side "b" specifically torn out. In my copy folio page 17 had the entire folio torn out, both sides "a" and "b." Most likely, this happened I feel because the recipe and its drawings were requested by a patient in distress who might have been on their way to see a doctor for relief. Such would indicate that my copy was being put to use by someone who valued its contents.

The set of these remedies were reprinted many times and offered to the public. In the reprinted versions available to the public, each publisher tried to distinguish their own version by altering the collection's title. For example, an 1892 edition was titled *Expanded Elaborations on the Seventy-Four Medical Therapies; Appendix of Forty Miraculous Old Therapies* (*Xinzeng xiuxiang qishisi fanzheng; houfu miaofang sishi yizhong* 新增繡像七十四翻症；後附妙方四十遺種, Damingtang *zi* 大明堂梓). It was for sale on the Chinese Kongfz.com website in 2021. The word *zi* 梓 indicates that this book publisher (the Damingtang) held the actual woodblocks. Putting the number seventy-four in the title allows us to conjecture that this publisher was not only reprinting the set, but had added to it.[35]

In comparing the texts of various online versions in relation to the contents of my own copy, I found that all versions were rather similar; they usually retained the same title for the disease, the presenting symptoms did not vary, and each recipe among the various printed sets recommended basically the same herbal ingredients. Most publishers respected the importance of the information being conveyed and they kept their editions faithful to the prior editions they used as a template. The differences in the content among the reprinted prescriptions were usually only minor changes in the wording used to express the individual recipes, and in the style of the illustrations. Some of the sets issued around 1916 had simple punctuation added in the recipes.

The Quirks in My Copy

My conclusion that the edition of my collection was circulating in the 1860s was determined by the illustrations of patients in distress appearing on each page. In a number of the similar volumes available online, those line drawings of other versions are clear and well-executed with strong lines in a presentation very different from the style used in my copy. Most of the lithographed editions from 1916, a year in which several publishing houses in China issued copies of this title, had drawings made by a professional artist. The bodies of those suffering from an affliction were clearly drawn, in proper proportions, and with some details as to the clothing they are wearing. By contrast, the line drawings in my copy are much simplified, with the thin lines of people in distress composed in a more abstract and impressionistic style. We have no clear illustration of the clothing they are wearing, or their expressions, or what historical period they might be from. If the illustrator of my edition was also a professional, they appear to have been working quickly and were not intent on conveying details. This was true both for the drawings of the associated animals and for the patient suffering the affliction.

Another book in my collection of old woodblock editions, on a different topic, helped me to determine the probable date of my copy of the *Seventy-Two Therapies*. I had purchased another book with illustrations that appeared to have been done by the same artist who did my copy of the medical manual. The drawing style is similar on many points and very different from the later twentieth-century lithographed reprints. The illustrations done in a similar style appear in a woodblock book titled *Pocket Edition of Precious Accurate Information; Imperial Calendar Almanac (Xiuli Jinbaizhongjing; Yuding wannianli* 袖裏金百中經；御定萬年曆). The calendar section in this almanac covers the years 1848 to 1864. The final pages are missing, but these dates tell me this edition was probably printed in 1848 and was very likely still circulating in 1864. I surmise the artist who made those drawings for the almanac in the mid-1800s was the same person who illustrated my edition of the *Seventy-Two Therapies*. It was common for Chinese almanacs to publish calendars of daily auspicious and inauspicious days for a period of years in advance so that it could be used to decide on dates for family and business affairs such as planning a wedding, arranging a funeral ceremony, or opening a new business. It would seem likely that the artist who illustrated the almanac published in 1848 was still alive in the 1860s. I also assume my manual was circulating in the markets then.

The first copy of the *Seventy-Two Therapies* was published in 1847 and the almanac I used was published in 1848, so it is possible the same artist was active at the times and was hired to contribute to both titles. Even if my copy of these remedies had come out in 1848, it is easy to assume it was still circulating in the 1860s, which is my more cautious estimate of its date.

Among the differences in the illustrated versions of the *Seventy-Two Therapies* available that I found while searching online was the differing order in which the therapies were presented. I had assumed each therapy was always presented in the same fixed order. But I found that the illnesses were arranged in differing sequences in the different versions. The way this happened is very easy to understand. In Chinese woodblock manufacture, each side of the woodblock almost always contained two pages. In that case the sheet of printed paper was meant to be folded vertically in the middle; it would be bound in string on the right-hand side, with the page number given along the middle fold. The center of the woodblock where the middle fold (*fengbu* 縫

部) appeared was called the fishtail (*yuwei* 魚尾). The term was a reference for the design typically used for the folded section of a single woodblock-printed sheet, seen in the illustration below.[36]

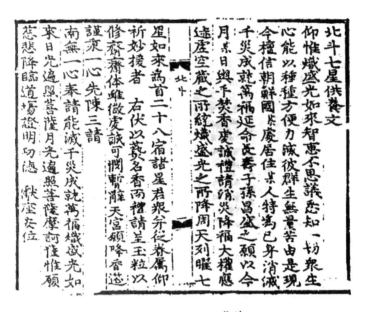

Page 1 in the section of the *Big Dipper* (*beidou* 北斗). The book's name is near the upper fishtail, the page number (one, 一) near the lower fishtail. This was the area of the outer fold. To our right is side "a," and to our left is side "b."

The result would be that each folio page had side "a" and side "b." The sides can be referred to as "leaf a" and "leaf b." By this counting my edition has thirty-nine pages with two sides each, for a total of seventy-eight individual pages. Traditional string-bound (*xianding* 線定) Chinese publications were numbered in this way.

When different editions of the *Seventy-Two Therapies* were re-cut the woodblocks sometimes got mixed up, so the sets of two pages (on a single woodblock) might be numbered in different sequences by the various woodblock cutters. This could happen because the individual therapies were not assigned any sequential identifier. In comparing my copy with several other illustrated online versions, I found that often the order of presentation was different while the order of each two sequential recipes, i.e. those on the same single sheet of woodblock printed paper, remained the same.

The therapies that appear in this translation follow the order as they appear in my copy of the *Seventy-Two Therapies*. I have numbered each therapy in sequence and treat it as if it were on the single page of a sequentially numbered publication. They are sequentially numbered as page one (P1), page two (P2), etc. In this translation no reference is made to the original page and leaf series. However, on the page photos in this book that are taken from my copy, one can see part of the original woodblock page numbers in the folded fishtail (*yuwei* 魚尾) on many of the illustrations.

To make another point about the particular copy I own, I have concluded that my copy was intended to be a very inexpensive, flimsy version of the *Seventy-Two Therapies* booklets then circulating. In the process of making a new, smaller, and inexpensive version of this title, the artist of the manual translated here was hired to draw each page in black and white on a piece of paper of the intended size of the new book. The artist hired to do the drawings for my copy of the manual worked quickly. The illustrations are simply drawn with no attention to detail. The corresponding animals on the page are sketched with the minimum number of lines. The written characters used to give the presenting symptoms, the name of the therapy, and then the ingredients of the medicines used, were hastily written in a small size in a manner that was often not very clear. The small size of the characters caused many of the medical recipes to become blurred when they were inked and printed. It is not clear if the artist of the illustrations and the person who wrote the words for the presenting symptoms and the remedy were the same person, but it does appear that both the written calligraphy and the illustrations were hurriedly done.

Once the drawing and writing of each woodblock consisting of two pages was completed, the paper would be given to woodblock carvers who would paste the drawing on a piece of wood, then carve the drawing into the wood. The paper was placed on the wood face-down because the carving had to be a mirror image of the printed page that would result. The artist's drawing could be easily seen through the thin paper. Woodblock carvers likely were semi-literate people who carved what was written but did not have the education to make corrections if a miswriting was present. I conclude the carvers of my manual were in this category. They followed the hastily written characters of the artist, but were not able to be more exact or clear about whether or not the characters were correctly or clearly written; there are cases of incorrectly written or mistaken characters in my copy.

My copy has thirty-nine sheets of folio pages, meaning each single sheet is folded once, with the folded edge being the left-hand (outside) edge of the page. As mentioned above, each side of the folio page therefore would have side "a" and side "b." As you look at the illustrated pages in this book, keep in mind that the Chinese book was opened from left to right and was read in vertical columns from top to bottom and from right to left. On the thirty-nine sheets of folio pages, there are sixty-four sides (pages) of printed material. As discussed above, among the pages illustrating specific therapies, a number of pages have disappeared, so my copy has an incomplete set of the therapies that originally appeared in this volume.

Handmade paper from the time, including my copy of the manual, tended to be of a brownish color because of the bamboo or rice straw used in its manufacture. It is very pliable, like a piece of cloth, and lightweight. It was stronger than it looked and, unlike machine-made paper, it did not easily tear. Further, it took the ink nicely without any blurring, and after these some 160 years since it was printed, the images are still very clear and the ink remains strongly black.

On a number of illustrated pages from my copy of the manual, you will see a stamp with the name Hao Liugui 郝留桂. This was an owner of my copy at some point in its life. I do not have information about this person. It would be wonderful if I could meet the previous owner of this manual to learn exactly how it was used. On the illustration of P23 and P36 you will see a stamp with the name Xue Long 薛龍; that is my Chinese name.

On the Word "Therapy"

One comment on the word I have translated in this manual as "therapy," "medical therapy," or "medical recipes." In pre-modern China it seems a colloquial word for "disease" was *fan* 翻. The word as used today means to "reverse" or to "overturn."[37] I assume this earlier usage of the word *fan* 翻 to mean a disease might have derived in spoken Chinese from the word for "trouble" (*mafan* 麻煩) which is written with different characters but might have been the basis for use of the word *fan* to mean disease. *Fan* 翻 for reverse is in the first tone, while *fan* 煩 for trouble is the second tone, so possibly my speculation is unfounded. When the word *fan* for "reverse" is coupled with the word for "illness" (*zheng* 症), as in the title of this collection, it could mean to reverse the illness, hence my translation of it as "therapy."[38] These treatments could also be called "remedies," "medical prescriptions," or "medical recipes."

The Doctor Approaches a Patient

When the Chinese doctor encountered a patient in distress, there were a number of actions an experienced doctor would take before proceeding with offering medication or relief. The first was to observe (*wang* 望) the person in distress to deduce as many characteristics of the patient and their situation as possible. The second was to take note (*wen* 聞) of the sound and smell of the patient. The third was when possible to ask (*wen* 問) the patient about how they felt, what they thought was causing their distress, and to receive if possible the patient's own view of their situation.[39] These were the basic actions to be performed upon initially meeting the patient. This could be followed by checking the tongue (*she* 舌) because the tongue relates to the meridians and organ systems throughout the body and indicates much about the conditions of the internal organs. There were, in addition, various physical appearances of the tongue noted by early Chinese researchers. Among these were fissures on the surface of the tongue (*sheche* 舌坼), stiffness at the base of the tongue (*shebenqiang* 舌本強), and dry (desiccated) tongue (*shegan* 舌乾).[40] The doctor could also tap various parts of the body along the meridians, or at the abdomen, or take the pulse of the patient. Only then would the doctor prescribe a medical course of action.[41]

These were the basic steps for all doctors or medical practitioners to follow before deciding on a treatment. The *Seventy-Two Therapies* is considered to have been for use in emergency situations when this methodical approach was not always possible so it does not make provision for the doctor's initial examination, nor does it give a detailed description of the patient. In this manual the set of presenting symptoms, taken together by the doctor, indicate the most likely effective therapy.

Medical Prescriptions

In a majority of cases in the collection of *Seventy-Two Therapies*, the prescription (*fangji* 方劑) involves herbal plants. The instructions given are to select particular herbs and grind them or burn them into a powder. In typical practice the medicinal powder was put in the mouth, followed by drinking a cup of a liquid. In most cases it is recommended the powder be ingested with yellow rice wine (*huangjiu* 黃酒), although sometimes tea or hot water are also recommended. In a very few cases cold water is recommended (P14, P18, P32). When the powder is mixed with the liquid and drunk we refer to it as a decoction (*tang* 湯), a word also used in Chinese to mean soup.

Alternatives to the basic recipe involving herbal plants were to use animal parts, such as the ground-down beak of a bird (P36, P37), or parts of a bird or insect nest (P35, P64d), etc. In some cases the powder resulting from burning an ingredient could be made into a pill (*wan* 丸; P29, P49), or into an ointment (*gao* 膏; P7, P12, P55, P57) to be rubbed on the affected part of the patient's body.[42] From my examination of various books of medical prescriptions, it appears that some practitioners preferred to prepare a pill, and less often a paste. But very often the type of decoction described in this manual was recommended. Was this because it perhaps suggested a degree of preparation and the ritual of drinking that had a positive psychological effect on the patient? Hand-written books of medical recipes available on the antiques markets in China in the early 2000s contained a preponderance of decoctions of the basic type of burnt herbs dissolved in a liquid.

The herbs prescribed were usually not harmful to the body, but we should keep in mind that the Chinese Pharmacopeia also included drugs that were poisonous (*du* 毒).[43] At times the prescription given in my manual could be accompanied by realgar, an arsenic sulfide mineral that occurs as crystals, or in a granular or powdery form, and is described in a number of the therapies, including the very first in this manual (P1). Realgar is toxic and poisonous, so it must be taken in small, controlled doses. Its Chinese name *xionghuang* 雄黃, literally meaning masculine yellow, an indication that it was considered very strong. It was a popular ingredient in the 1860s and in this manual it is prescribed sixteen times.[44] Highly toxic or poisonous ingredients were not often recommended by traditional Chinese medical practitioners, but they could provide a "jolt" to the system when needed, just as was the case with "striking" a patient as a way to shock the system back into more normal functioning.

The Chinese doctor consulting the *Seventy-Two Therapies* booklet in the 1860s used a measuring/weighing system handed down from earlier ages. As referenced in this translated manual and using the values prevalent in the late Qing and Republic, a *jin* 斤 is 570 grams or 1.316 pounds. The *liang* 兩 is

37.301 grams or 1.316 ounces. The *qian* 錢 (dividing the *liang* by 10) is 3.7301 grams or 0.1316 ounce. Note that the *qian* as it appears in the latter medical recipes in the collection translated here is written with a character often used by pharmacists in China in the 1860s as 亇. The *fen* 分 is a hundredth of a *liang*, or 373.01 milligrams or 0.01316 ounce.[45] These measurements also have European-influenced designations no longer in use: the *jin* was a catty, the *liang* was a tael, the *qian* was a mace, and the *fen* was a candareen.

The majority of therapies in this manual do not specify the amount of material to be used, although the final grouping of unillustrated maladies at the end of the manual contains amounts according to the measurement system described above. This change in the presentation of the therapies tells me that the latter unillustrated therapies were authored by a person different from the one who put together the basic set of this publication. A doctor or practitioner of folk medicine no doubt did not need precise measurements and assembled the ingredients in amounts based on their experience. Most of the 1916 reprints I have seen did not include measurements for the ingredients used. A general consensus among scholars is that Chinese medical practitioners in the nineteenth and early twentieth centuries did not use precise measurements when they prepared or administered decoctions.

A Closing Statement

I have added a short commentary to each of the recipes translated in this book. My purpose in the commentaries was to investigate if the herbs recommended in each therapy were likely to have a positive effect on the internal organs or physical conditions thought to be the cause of the affliction. I found that the ancient Chinese research into medical plants and herbs had been thorough, and the effectiveness of their suggested uses have been repeatedly confirmed by modern medical researchers using recent and scientifically rigorous research methods. This speaks well of the centuries of careful observation, experimentation, and record keeping that the Chinese scholars and medical practitioners followed. Their assumptions about how the human body worked and how the interactions of several factors affected human health were well-founded.

There are a few basic observations that have guided my work on the translation of this manual. First, the approaches to medical issues and the remedies offered to Chinese patients in this manual were in many ways not so different from those being offered in Western medicine at the time. For example, blood-letting as a way to relieve pressures within the body and remove pathogens was practiced in Western cultures and by the 1860s was still being prescribed. Today it is sometimes recommended in limited cases. In the late 1800s and early 1900s, in the United States many "patent medicines" and health tonics of unspecific ingredients were being sold to the public by traveling "medical doctors" as part of a medicine show. Buying a bottle of medicine or a good all-purpose tonic was often part of an entertainment performance offered in small, rural towns in the United States well into the 1920s. The joke mentioned by some people was that the alcohol contained in the medicine gave an "extra boost" to those who took the medicine, and raised the question asking if the medicine was in fact another way to indulge in alcohol consumption. These tonics sold in small towns of America were often jokingly referred to as "snake oil," a term which always draws to my mind the vendor displaying snakes and selling medicine I saw at an outdoor fair in Hangzhou in 2012.

Second, the traditional categories used by the Chinese to explain the causes and cures of ailments were as well-founded and inter-related as were those of Western medicine at the time. Medical theorists in Western cultures early described the four humors of Hippocratic medicine: black bile, yellow bile, phlegm, and blood. One can see a similarity to the idea of the energy of *qi* propelling blood through the channels, and the ways the fluid could become diseased and change color from red to purple or black. Today Western scientists say that the chemicals contained in bile help with the digestion of fats in the body, and they help to absorb fat-soluble vitamins such as A, D, E, and K. (I recognize that the chemical composition of the early Greek and current medical definitions of "bile" are likely to be different.) Nevertheless, such connections reinforce the idea of medical theory as a long-term continuous process evolving over centuries. Body temperature played a role in these bodily interactions in both the Western and Asian traditions. In the Asian approach, the influence of either heat or cold became the basis for influential theories of pathogenic disorders.

As we have seen thus far, enumerating the harmful effects of cold (*han* 寒) as a cause of a medical condition has been a major approach by Chinese doctors in classical Chinese medicine. But among Korean scholars, attention has also been given to the effect of excess heat (*re* 熱) as we see in some of the commentaries in this manual. Korean medical scholars have identified a syndrome labeled *hwabyung* 火病, which means "fire disease." Traditional Korean medicine explains that *hwabyung* is caused by suffering extreme psychological or emotional stress for a prolonged time. Chronic stress over activates heat (fire/anger), and accumulates in the heart, liver, stomach, head, or chest, which in turn provokes the *hwabyung*.

Some of the physical effects of *hwabyung* include "a stuffy feeling in the chest, frequent sighing, palpitations, fatigue, hot or cold sensations, heaviness of the head, insomnia, localized or generalized aches and pains, dry mouth, indigestion, anorexia, dizziness, nausea. . . ." Modern researchers define some of these symptoms as related to psychosomatic conditions such as "major depression, anxiety disorder, somatization disorder, panic disorder, posttraumatic stress disorder, phobic disorder, and obsessive-compulsive disorders."[46] The age-old medical theories appear to apply quite well to explain modern ailments.

The Chinese traditional theories of winds (*feng* 風), dampness (*shi* 濕), heat (*re* 熱), and the circulation of liquids within the body are an inter-connected way of explaining how the systems of the body operate. This manual was based on the theories that developed in the long flow of China's history and culture and will make logical sense to someone who has received a sudden chill from the wind or become ill from being over-dressed on a day the temperatures rise. These connections of temperature, wind, dampness, and heat seem to be accepted by a majority of human beings, even by those who do not know of the Asian theories of how they interact.

Third, the typical reader of these medical therapies going through my translations in contemporary times might feel some therapies are strange and maybe even suspect. Using cow dung, or slapping the patient's forehead? But current Western scientific methods show that the classical Chinese medical recipes offered in this manual were both based on centuries of careful observation and almost all of them have a chemical basis confirmed by research conducted along Western scientific methods. Case in point: recent research shows that chemicals in the grasshopper have anticancer effects (discussed in P26).[47] There are a number of similar examples in the translated folk remedies. This means that we are unwise to arbitrarily reject the medical prescriptions in the manual as ill-founded. The ingredients suggested in these therapies were easily available to most people in rural China, and represented a way of using naturally-occurring plants and herbs to provide healing.

In closing this Introduction, I wish to state that the information in this book is offered as historical interest, as a way to reconstruct something of the world of the Chinese people around 1860. The common people of the time, in need of medical attention, were likely to bring their affliction to a medical practitioner, who was likely to have consulted a version of this handy and popular manual. My translation is not intended to offer medical advice. I hope it will offer respect for China's long tradition of medical research and will excite an interest in the reader to learn more about folk remedies in old China.

Notes

1   A useful and comprehensive explanation of China's history of medical thinking and its applications to recurring illnesses is Liu Lihong, *Classical Chinese Medicine* (Hong Kong: The Chinese University Press, 2019). The text is clear and easy to follow and many of the details of how medical concepts were formed are given. An insightful study of classical Chinese medical thought and that of Greek civilization is Sigehisa Kuriyama, *The Expressiveness of the Body and the Divergence of Greek and Chinese Medicine* (Princeton, NJ: Princeton University Press, 1999).

2   The Chinese language version of this paragraph reads: "《七十二翻》是中醫治療急證險證的經典文獻,其文字圖形簡單到不能再簡單的地步。其包含的醫理卻深不見底。中醫認為,每一種疾病都有特定的病理敏感點、顯露點、對應點,找到這些點及時有效地加以處理,便能救人於頃刻之間。中醫的挑治療法、火針療法、巨針療法看似殘酷,那是救命的絕活。從古至今不知挽回多少人的生命。切要重視。" From http://blog.sina.com.cn/s/blog_513a59070102vds1. html, accessed July 2021. The two therapies mentioned in this description for acupuncture treatments are actually not mentioned in most collections of the *Seventy-Two Therapies*. Note that the Hot Needle and Large Needle therapies were not included in my copy of the manual translated here.

3   In addition to the basic approach of burning the herbs into a powder and having the patient ingest them with tea or wine, several other techniques to be used in treating the patient are recommended in this translated manual. Among them are the following: hitting or striking (*da* 打) the patient, P1, P4,

P8, P59; using bird or insect nests, P35, P64d; making a pill (*wan* 丸), P29, P49; preparing an ointment (*gao* 膏), P7, P12, P55, P57; using animal fecal matter or animal dung, P25, P61c; using tobacco tar (*yanyou* 煙油), P7, P16, P51; using human or animal urine, P26, P61d, P64a. Several recipes suggesting the use of human or animal waste are quoted in Paul U. Unschuld, *Traditional Chinese Medicine: Heritage and Adaptation* (New York: Columbia University Press, 2018), pp. 109–110. Also see Huan Du et al., "Fecal Medicines Used in Traditional Medical System of China: A Systematic Review of Their Names, Original Species, Traditional Uses, and Modern Investigations," *Chinese Medicine* 14.31 (September 2019), DOI: 10.1186/s13020-019-0253-x.

4   See Otsuka Keisetsu 大塚敬節 et al., *Kanpō dai'iten* 漢方大医典 (Dictionary of Chinese Medicine) (Tokyo: Tōto shobō 東都書房, 1957). In particular see the section on "Popular Medicine" (*minkanyaku* 民間藥) by Kurihara Hirozo 栗原広三, pp. 86–88. This section describes how the remedies would be prepared even in the home. It was important to usually wash the plants, keeping the water clear, and using an earthen pot if possible, never a metal cooking utensil. Small amounts were adequate, perhaps 600 cc. or 20.2 ounces (about two cups) of water, which would be reduced during the boiling process. Explanations of collecting and preparing traditional medicines are in Daegu Yangnyeongsi Oriental Medicine Museum 大邱藥令市韓醫藥博物館 website, https://daegu. go.kr/dgom. Illustrated pamphlets are available in Chinese, Japanese, and English versions. The Museum has dioramas of both collecting and selling these herbs in traditional times, and the city still maintains a public herbal market.

5   The close relationship between these medical recipes and self-administered medicine among the common people is mentioned several times by Unschuld, *Traditional Chinese Medicine.* By the late Qing period, Chinese doctors offering traditional medicine in China's largest cities were advertising in the local periodical press. Some of their advertisements are reprinted in Rachel Silberstein, *A Fashionable Century: Textile Artistry and Commerce in the Late Qing* (Seattle, WA: University of Washington Press, 2020). See p. 175, the five ads of the left-hand side. The ads are read from right to left.

6   The manual translated here contains simple, basic recipes because it was intended for emergency use. Chinese medical practitioners seem to have expected there would be times calling for immediate care. In fact, the specific recommendation given in such situations was "When urgent, treat the symptoms first" (*ji, ze zhi qi biao* 急，則治其標). See *Huangdi Neijing: A Synopsis with Commentaries* (*Neijing zhiyao yigu* 內經知要譯詁), trans. and annot. Y. C. Kong (Kong Yun-cheung 江潤祥) (Hong Kong: The Chinese University Press, 2010), p. 452.

7   The book by Liu Lihong, *Classical Chinese Medicine*, is an example of how medicine was studied based on well-established texts and would be explained by a highly literate and well-educated practitioner. This text draws heavily on China's historical record to explain how medical thinking is applied when approaching various maladies.

8   Several English language translations of the *Yellow Emperor's Classic* are available. The book mentioned in an earlier endnote above, *Huangdi Neijing: A Synopsis with Commentaries*, is as its title indicating a rather scholarly and highly annotated version. There are friendlier versions in English. One of those is a partial translation titled *The Yellow Emperor's Classic of Internal Medicine*, translated by Ilza Veith (Berkeley, CA: University of California Press, 2002). This translation focuses on the Basic Questions (*suwen* 素問) portion of the classic and gives the foundational principles and theoretical thinking of the *Yellow Emperor's Classic*. Her translation was initially published in 1949. A work that discusses and gives classificatory points on the contents of the Basic Questions is Iemoto Sei'ichi 家本誠一, *Outline of Chinese Classical Medicine: The Origins of Herbal Medicine and Acupuncture* (*Chūgoku kodai igaku taikei: Kanpō, shinkyū no genryū* 中国古代医学大系：漢方鍼灸の源流) (Tokyo: Seifūsha 靜風社, 2017). See pp. 427–453.

9   Vivienne Lo, "Imagining Practice: Sense and Sensuality in Early Chinese Medical Illustration," Chapter 3, in Vivienne Lo et al., *Imagining Chinese Medicine* (Leiden: Brill, 2018), p. 75.

10 The *Yellow Emperor's Classic* is composed of two sections, the first being the Basic Questions (*suwen* 素問) which lays out the fundamental thinking about drug and herbal interactions. The second is the Spiritual Hinge (*lingshu* 靈樞, sometimes translated as the Numinous Pivot) that delves into acupuncture therapy. As Chinese medical and cosmological theories were being developed in the Han Dynasty, they often included the idea of a center point around which forces and changes coalesced, even if only temporarily, in order to radiate outward again. A detailed discussion of the Spiritual Hinge is in Mayanagi Makoto 直柳誠, *Research on the Yellow Emperor's Medical Texts* (*Kōtei iseki kenkyū* 黄帝医籍研究) (Tokyo: Kyūko shoin 汲古書院, 2014). See Chapter Two, pp. 189–259.

11 A thoughtful reinterpretation of the intellectual basis for Chinese cosmological and medical thinking, translated from German, is Paul U. Unschuld, *Traditional Chinese Medicine*. He has published a number of books about Chinese medicine and many of his ideas are at the forefront of current Western thinking about this topic. Another overall review of Chinese medical thinking and approaches, this version accepting all traditionally held Chinese views, is Heinrich Wallnofer and

Anna Von Rottauscher, *Chinese Folk Medicine* (New York: Bell Publishing, 1965), translated from the German by Marion Palmedo.

12 It is often stated that the term TCM (Traditional Chinese Medicine) was devised by scholars in the People's Republic of China in 1955 as a way to elevate Chinese traditional medical practices to the status of a formal body of medical knowledge. The origin of the term is thus seen as having been largely political in nature. See the discussions in Unschuld, *Traditional Chinese Medicine*; and Liu Lihong, *Classical Chinese Medicine*, particularly the Introduction by Heiner Fruehauf, pp. xix–xlv.

13 An outline of Ayurveda practices is given in a posting about dealing with cancer in "Ayurvedic Medicine," *Cancer Research UK*, accessed April 18, 2022. The organization's website is https://www.cancerresearchuk.org/.

14 On Hua Tuo, see Victor Mair, "The Biography of Hua-t'o from the 'History of the Three Kingdoms,'" in Victor H. Mair (ed.), *The Columbia Anthology of Traditional Chinese Literature* (New York: Columbia University Press, 1994), pp. 688–696.

15 Copies of Zhang's work as collected by students were later published. One of the most well-known has been put out in a facsimile edition in Japan. This is the title *Annotations of the Theory of Febrile Diseases* (*Zhujie Shanghanlun* 注解傷寒論). The version published is a Yuan 元 Dynasty edition that had been compiled by Cheng Wuji 成無己 (1063–1156) in the Jin 金 Dynasty (1115–1234). This appears in the series *Collection of Rare Books on Asian Medicine, Volume Two* (*Tōhō igaku zenhon sōkan, dainisaku* 東方医学善本叢刊，第二冊 (Osaka: Oriento shuppansha, 2001). Cheng's work has been translated into English as Jonathan Schell, trans., *Discussion of Cold Damage with Annotations* (Portland, OR: Chinese Medicine Database, 2018).

16 See Hsu Hong-Yen et al., ed., *Shang Han Lun* (*The Great Classic of Chinese Medicine*) (Los Angeles: Oriental Healing Arts Institute, 1981). In this book, Zhang's name is given as Chang Chung-Ching, reflecting the Wade-Giles romanization system used at the time. A woodblock edition in my collection is *Precious Imperial Compendium of the Medical Profession, Vol. 17: Revised Annotations on Cold Injuries* (*Yuzuan yicong jinjian, juan shiqi: Dingzheng Shanghanlun zhu zhengwu pian* 御纂醫宗金鑒，卷十七：訂正傷寒論註正誤篇) in the *Siku quanshu* 四庫全書 finally issued in 1793. This title became the standard reference work for all doctors in north China. This is a woodblock version of Volume 17 with many pages missing. Size is 4 ⅞ inch (12.4 cm) w. × 7 ⅝ inch (19.4 cm) h.

17 The ways in which both traditional and current concepts and observations are applied in Chinese medicine are given detailed explanations in Nigel Wiseman and Andrew Ellis, *Fundamentals of Chinese Medicine, Revised Edition* (Brookline, MA, 1995). This is a complete translation of the standard reference work *Zhongyixue jichu* 中醫學基礎, published in China in 1985.

18 Many legends have grown up around Sun Simiao. "Once he extracted a bone that had been caught in a tiger's gullet and in gratitude the tiger became his protector. Sun's image is often with a tiger close by or he is riding on a tiger. Another time he rescued the son of the Dragon King from a beating given by a shepherd. As a reward the Dragon King gave him a book on medicine. . . ." See Anne S. Goodrich, *Peking Paper Gods: A Look at Home Worship* (Nettetal: Steyler Verlag, 1991), p. 140. Indeed, most votive images or statues of Sun depict him with a tiger, a dragon, and sometimes holding a needle, in reference to ideas of acupuncture.

19 These three have been selected by the Daoists at Baiyunguan as the most important Kings of Medicine, but others have also been so named in popular culture. For an example, see *True Classic of the Lingying Medicine King* (*Lingying yaowang zhenjing* 靈應藥王真經). This edition published in 2014 by the Saiwudang Daoists Association of Taishan Monastery in Shiyan city, Hubei province 湖北省十堰市賽武當協泰山觀. The text was compiled by Qin Yue 秦越 during the Warring States period (475–221 BCE). This locally famous hero devised effective medicines.

20 A very useful publication describing herbal plants used for medical purposes is *Dictionary of the Ben Cao Gang Mu, Volume I: Chinese Historical Illness Terminology*, ed. Zhang Zhibin and Paul U. Unschuld (Oakland, CA: University of California Press, 2015). This is an important and carefully prepared translation of the classic often rendered in English as *Compendium of Materia Medica* (*Bencao gangmu* 本草綱目). Interesting comments on the strong and less strong points of this compendium are given in Nicholas K. Menzies, *Ordering the Myriad Things: From Traditional Knowledge to Scientific Botany in China* (Seattle: University of Washington Press, 2021). The development of a pharmacopia in China through the use of testing and classifying herbs is in Bian He 邊和 (publishing in English as He Bian), *Know Your Remedies: Pharmacy and Culture in Early Modern China* (Princeton, NJ: Princeton University Press, 2020). A contemporary explanation of commonly used medical herbs in Taiwan is in Deng Huichun 鄧慧純, "Have You Had Your Herbs Today?: Welcome to the World of Taiwanese Herbs," *Taiwan Panorama* (April 2023): 76–87. The article is bilingual in Chinese and English.

21 The historical flow of information between China, Central Asia, and the West, including advances concerning medicine and pharmacology, are described in Pamela Kyle Crossley, *Hammer and Anvil: Nomad Rulers at the Forge of the Modern World* (London: Rowman & Littlefield, 2019). An account of medicinal herbs known and used in South Siberia/North Manchuria, and investigated by Russian botanists, is in Ruth Rogaski, *Knowing Manchuria: Environments, the Senses, and Natural Knowledge on an Asian Borderland* (Chicago: University of Chicago Press, 2022), Chapter 4.

22 Treating the highest elites in Korea, the king and his relatives, with herbal medicine, was inserted into official records of the Korean government during the 1600s and 1700s. See *The King's Mouthpiece: Institute for the Translation of Korean Classics,* trans. Yi-Yung Kim (Seoul: Jipmoondang, 2019), pp. 110, 170. These are selected translations with contemporary commentaries of the Diaries of the Royal Secretariat (*Sŭngjŏngwŏn ilgi* 승정원 일기, 承政院日記) from the Joseon period (1392–1910). When an illness flared, the person stricken or their relatives in Korea might have also turned to Buddhist teaching, since Buddhism was widely practiced. Equally, they may have turned to a local shaman (*mudang* 무당, 巫堂) since shamanic beliefs in the prevalence of spirits in all things was part of age-old practices among the Koreans. These are vividly described in all the works by cultural anthropologist Laurel Kendall, including *Mediums and Magical Things: Statues, Paintings, and Masks in Asian Places* (Oakland, CA: University of California Press, 2022).

23 See Hoang Bao Chau and Pho Duc Thuc, et al., *Vietnamese Traditional Medicine* (Hanoi: The Gioi [World] Publishers, 2016). This work lists many medical recipes based on traditional folk medicine, with an obvious influence from Chinese traditional medical practices.

24 The character meaning needle (*zhen* 針) was traditionally written 鍼, which is how it appears in historical texts. The theoretical and philosophical basis of acupuncture is explained in Yang Zhenhai 楊真海, *The Yellow Emperor's Inner Transmission of Acupuncture* (*Huangdi neizhen* 黃帝內針), trans. Sabine Wilms (Hong Kong: The Chinese University of Hong Kong Press, 2020).

25 The channels are also referred to as blood vessels, or as a pulse. An excellent discussion of these terms is in Vivienne Lo, "Imagining Practice: Sense and Sensuality in Early Chinese Medical Illustration," in Lo et al., *Imagining Chinese Medicine*, pp. 69–88. Some Chinese scholars distinguish between the channels that carried blood, and the channels that carried the vital energy force of *qi* 氣, but it is difficult to clearly define how the two systems differed or exactly where in the body they were located. A review of research on this point will reveal

the absence of universally accepted agreement about the differences between channels and meridians.

26 A detailed, working manual about acupuncture is Andrew Ellis, Nigel Wiseman, Ken Boss, and James Cleaver, *Fundamentals of Chinese Acupuncture, Revised Edition* (Taos, NM: Paradigm Publications, 2004). A lithographed edition of a woodblock publication in my collection dealing specifically with pustules is *Essential for Treating Pustules* (*Zhiding yaoshu* 治疗要書) (Shanghai: Hongda shanshuju 宏大善書局, 1927). From the many times these discolorations (*ding* 疔) are mentioned in the manual translated here, I conclude these were a common problem in old China. They were easy to see and were visible indications of a medical condition requiring treatment.

27 Comments on the early use of needles and "blood-letting" are in T. J. Hinrichs and Linda L. Barnes, *Chinese Medicine and Healing: An Illustrated History* (Cambridge, MA: Harvard University Press, 2013), pp. 200, 234.

28 A discussion about the exact or non-exact location of acupuncture points is in Yang Zhenhai 楊真海, *The Yellow Emperor's Inner Transmission of Acupuncture* (*Huangdi neizhen* 黃帝內針), pp. 35, 97–134. Note that Yang references a different system of assigning numbers to the meridians and acupuncture points than is given in my book.

29 The Pool at the Bend (*quchixue* 曲池穴) is mentioned in P2 and P38.

30 For an explanation of this point, see *Dictionary of Chinese Traditional Health* (*Zhongguo chuantong yangshengxue cidian* 中國傳統養生學辭典), ed. Zhuang Huafeng 莊華峰 and Fang Baiying 方百盈 (Nanning: Guangxi jiaoyu chubanshe 廣西教育出版社, 1996), p. 727.

31 The case of a serious and well-trained medical doctor who also would prescribe Daoist incantations and rituals to scare away the demons which brought sickness is discussed in Ronald Suleski, *Daily Life for the Common People of China, 1850 to 1950: Understanding* Chaoben *Culture* (Leiden: Brill, 2018). See the comments about Dr. He Jinliang 何錦樑 in Chapter 3, pp. 134–140. The link between gods, spirits, and demons is explored in Michel Strickmann and Barnard Faure, eds., *Chinese Magical Medicine* (Stanford, CA: Stanford University Press, 2002). An actual example of the acknowledgement of demons and medical knowledge by the people who were listening to a popular story from China's past is in Kristin Ingrid Fryklund, trans., *The Lady of Linshui Pacifies Demons: A Seventeenth-Century Novel* (Seattle: University of Washington Press, 2021). The novel's original title is *Linshui pingyao* 臨水平妖. In Chapter 7, p. 86, the demons act according to the idea that "pressing the pulses gives access to all the organs of the body for

diagnoses, or allows the taking possession of the body if one is a ritual master (*fashi* 法士)." This explanation given on p. 266.

32 See Chu Ping-Yi (Zhu Pingyi 祝平一), "Qingdai de shazheng: Yige jibing fanchou de dansheng" 清代的痧症：一個疾病範疇的誕生 (Cholera in the Qing Dynasty: The Birth of a Disease Category), *Hanxue yanjiu* 漢學研究 (*Chinese Studies*) 31.3 (September 2014).

33 *Headaches* (*Toutong* 頭痛 / *touteng* 頭疼). This is a hand-written manual in my collection likely written by an acupuncturist for his own use. It is filled with line drawings of the human body, each page illustrating the areas where needles could be inserted to treat particular conditions such as toothache (*yateng* 牙疼), lack of breast milk in a nursing woman (*furen wu nai* 婦人無奶), unable to move the feet (*zu bu neng xing* 足不能行), etc. It appears this was written by a Mr. Liu 劉氏, the owner of the Zhengdetang 政德堂, probably a pharmacy (*yaoju* 藥局) in Shandong 山東, Jiaozhou-fu 交州府, Taizhuang 台莊, Chengnan 城南. Probably written in the late Qing. A page from this book is illustrated in Appendix B.

34 As part of my research, I have been trying to identify various editions and versions of this title. Comments on the versions I have located are given in the publication history of this title in Appendix A.

35 The differing titles and related editions circulated in various formats are discussed in Appendix A. The research I did online would be usefully complemented by a search of library collections in order to see which editions are held by libraries.

36 This is a Daoist religious text discussing worship of the Big Dipper (*beidou* 北斗), which is composed of seven stars. The illustration is labeled: "Ritual text for veneration of the Big Dipper (K. *Bukduchilseong gongyangmun*), Published at Ssanggyesa Temple, Eunjin, Joseon (1580), 19.2 × 11.5 cm, Gapsa Temple. Source: (Park 1987, p. 179)." This illustration was taken from Kim Jahyun, "Korean Single-Sheet Buddhist Woodblock Illustrated Prints Produced for Protection and Worship," *Religions* 11.12 (2020): 647, https://doi.org/10.3390/rel11120647.

37 The idea of using this word in its broader sense is explained in *Comprehensive Chinese-English Dictionary* (*Han-Ying zonghe da cidian* 漢英綜合大辭典), ed. Wu Guanghua (Dalian: Ligong daxue chubanshe 理工大學出版社, 2004); see pp. 1231, 1229. It defines the word *fan* 翻 as meaning repent, change, correct, and restore. It uses the phrase "change the bad into good, change evil into orthodox" (*gaie huishan, gaixie guizheng* 改惡回善，改邪歸正). In this thinking,

the word therapy (*fanzheng* 翻症) could be said to mean "reversing" (*fan* 翻) the "disease" or "affliction" (*zheng* 症). Treatment to cure a disease would be a "therapy."

38 The popular usage of the word *fan* 翻 was to mean a disease. It also had reference to intervention in "medical emergencies or crisis situations" (*luanweiji jieduan* 亂危急階段), or "medical situations bringing on a fever (febrile disease)" (*wenbing* 溫病). Commentary pointing to these cases is in *Medical Literature* (*Zhongyi wenxian* 中醫文獻), ed. Chen Rong 陳榮 et al. (Beijing: Zhongyi guji chubanshe 中醫古籍出版社, 2007), Vol. 2, p. 1253. This interpretation is reinforced by the explanation of the *Seventy-Two Therapies* given in *Chinese Dictionary of Medical Books* (*Zhongguo yiji da cidian* 中國醫籍大辭典), ed. the Compilation Committee (*Bianzuan weiyuanhui* 編纂委員會) (Shanghai: Shanghai Scientific Press [*Shanghai kexue jishu chubanshe* 上海科學技術出版社], 2002), Vol. 1, p. 744. In this title, see HO 445 for a definition of the *Seventy-Two Therapies*. In defining the book *Considering Therapies: Illustrated* (*Fanzheng tukao* 翻症圖考), it says the word *fanzheng* 翻症 (therapies) actually refers to the "symptoms of convulsions and wind present in the critical stages of cholera" (*huoluan weiji jieduan chuxian chouchu dongfeng zhengzhuang, chengzhi fanzheng* 霍亂危急階段出現抽搐動風症狀，稱之翻症).

39 Bao Jinjian 寶金劍, ed., *Cartoon TCM, Vol. 5: Medical Prescriptions* (*Zhongyi manhua, di-wu ce: Fangji* 中醫漫畫，第五冊：方劑) (Beijing: Zhongguo kexue jishu chubanshe 中國科學技術出版社, 2018), p. 1. This title uses a comic book format to present a number of medical conditions affecting the internal organs as taken from the Basic Questions (*suwen* 素問) section of the *Yellow Emperor's Classic*. In regard to the importance of centering on the patient and their affliction, see Liu Bangming 劉幫明, *Inspection of Face and Body for Diagnosis of Diseases*, 2nd ed. (Beijing: Foreign Languages Press, 2006). This is an English language translation of *Chayan guanse cebaibing* 察顏觀色測百病 published in 2002. The face reveals much about the individual. It is used to predict one's fate and future when employed in fortunetelling (*mianxiang* 面相). Medical practitioners in China noted conditions of the face, such as facial gloom (*miangan* 面玕), facial blisters (*mianpao* 面皰), and clogged-up facial sores (*mianyanchuang* 面涇瘡). See *Dictionary of the Ben Cao Gang Mu, Volume I*, pp. 340–341.

40 The importance of the tongue (*she* 舌) in the recommended therapies is specified in: P5, P10, P14, P16, P39, P41, P49, P50, P51, and P53. Additional physical manifestations of the tongue are listed in *Dictionary of the Ben Cao Gang Mu, Volume I*, pp. 430–438. Among the common conditions noted are purple tongue (*shezi* 舌紫), tongue swelling (*shezhong* 舌腫), and tongue fur (*shetai* 舌胎).

41 In my personal collection is a woodblock edition of *Precious Imperial Compendium of the Medical Profession, Vol. 3: Correct Procedures in External Medicine for the Heart-Mind* (*Yuzuan yicong jinjian, juan san: Bianji waike xinfa yaojue* 御纂醫宗金鑒, 卷三：編輯外科心法要訣). The entire set consisted of ninety volumes. It was included in the massive Qing project of the Imperial Library in Four Sections (*Siku quanshu* 四庫全書) finally issued in 1793. This Volume Three deals with external medicine and the basic steps the doctor goes through in externally examining the patient and considering a prescription. 4 ⅞ inch (12.4 cm) w. × 7 ⅝ inch (19.4 cm) h.

42 The various ways of delivering medical prescriptions were through decoctions (*tang* 湯), pills (*wan* 丸), powders (*san* 散), pastes (*gao* 膏), syrups (*lu* 露), or wine (*jiu* 酒), as discussed in Bao Jinjian, *Cartoon TCM, Vol. 5*, pp. 122–129. A good description of pastes is in *Basic Chinese Medical Dictionary* (*Jianming Zhongyi zidian* 簡明中醫字典), ed. Yang Huasen 楊華森 et al. (Guiyang: Guizhou renmin chubanshe 貴州人民出版社, 1985), p. 410.

43 An excellent study on the use of strong herbs and minerals in the delivery of curative medical prescriptions is Yan Liu, *Healing with Poisons: Potent Medicines in Medieval China* (Seattle, WA: Washington University Press, 2021). The logic was that a fierce pathogen needed strong medicine to dislodge it. A touch of realgar in a typical decoction would also have that effect.

44 Prescribing the use of realgar (*xionghuang* 雄黃) in a medical recipe is recommended in this manual sixteen times: P1, P2, P14, P15, P17, P18, P32, P40, P41, P42, P43, P44, P46, P49, P53, and P60.

45 Bao Jinjian, *Cartoon TCM, Vol. 5*, pp. 114–121. A brief mention of amounts used, cited above, is in Otsuka Keisetsu 大塚敬節 et al., *Kanpō dai'iten* 漢方大医典 (Dictionary of Chinese Medicine) (Tokyo: Tōto shobō 東都書房, 1957). In particular, see the section on "Popular Medicine" (*minkanyaku* 民間藥) by Kurihara Hirozo 栗原広三, pp. 86–88. Weight equivalencies in the Qing are listed in Bao Xiangao 鮑相璈, *Raising the Dead and Returning Life: Emergency Medicine of the Qing Dynasty* (*Qisi huisheng* 起死回生), trans. Lorraine Wilcox (Portland, OR: Chinese Medical Database, 2012), p. 20. These lists of equivalencies and those mentioned in my Introduction do not agree precisely but they do in general. Current research on traditional methods for dealing with injuries to the body is being carried out by Professor Yi-Li Wu at the University of Michigan in her study *The Injured Body: A Social History of Medicine for Wounds in Late Imperial China* (forthcoming).

46 For a contemporary evaluation of this affliction, see Jonghyun Lee, "*Hwabyung* and Depressive Symptoms among Korean Immigrants," *Social Work in Mental Health* 13.2 (2015): 159–185, DOI: 10.1080/15332985.2013.812538.

47 The typical word in Chinese for a grasshopper is *zhàměng* 蚱蜢. In P26 of the
Seventy-Two Therapies, the word used is *jila* 虮蜡 (which can also be written as 蟣
蠟). The term might be broadly defined as the mucus or sticky substance taken
from an insect. For the past several decades, medical researchers in China have
been keen to find linkages between traditional Chinese medical ingredients and
medical effectiveness based on Western scientific research.

THE SEVENTY-TWO THERAPIES

QISHIER FANZHENG

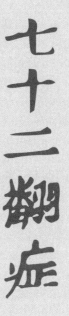

P1. Phoenix Therapy
Fenghuang zhanchi fan zhi 鳳凰展翅翻治

Presenting Symptom: The Arms Flap.

Qi xing: Gugong yaobai.

其形：股肱搖擺。

Phoenix Therapy. Strike the palm and waist with the sole of a shoe to relieve symptoms. After that, drink realgar water.

Fenghuang zhanchi fan zhi. Yong xiedi da shouxin yu yao, zai yi xionghuangshui yin zhi.

鳳凰展翅翻治。用鞋底打手心與腰，再以雄黃水飲之。

This is called Phoenix Therapy because the patient's arms extend like wings and flap against the thigh. A Western medical term for this would be asterixis, a clinical sign that describes the inability to maintain sustained posture, often with subsequent brief, shock-like, involuntary movements. A reference to arms flapping as a symptom of a disease is: R. Nayak et al., "Asterixis (Flapping Tremors) As an Outcome of Complex Psychotropic Drug Interaction," *Journal of Neuropsychiatry and Clinical Neuroscience* 24.1 (Winter 2012): 27–29.

Note that the title of this therapy could also be translated as Phoenix Extended Wings Therapy (*Fenghuang zhanchi fan* 鳳凰展翅翻).

To the Chinese practitioner, this flapping tremor indicated a serious underlying disease process. Most likely the shoe referred to here had a cotton cloth sole, and the slap would not result in a bruise. For more on the recommendation of hitting, see P4 below. At least eleven of the therapies in this manual recommend hitting.

Realgar (*xionghuang* 雄黃) is an arsenic sulfide mineral. It is bitter, acrid, and toxic. It was usually ground into a fine powder and mixed with water or yellow rice wine (*huangjiu* 黃酒), to be drunk. Among its perceived uses at the time, realgar was believed to repel harmful creatures and spirits, so people drank realgar wine during the Dragon Boat Festival (*duanwujie* 端午節, on the fifth day of the fifth month of the Chinese calendar, which corresponds to late May or June in the Gregorian calendar) to expel devils. In Chinese medicine realgar has been used for the treatment of both internal and external diseases such as infection, inflammation, fever, convulsion, and even some skin diseases. In recent times it has been used to combat the spread of cancer because it acts to inhibit the proliferation of diseased cells in the blood. Several other therapies in this manual prescribe the use of realgar.

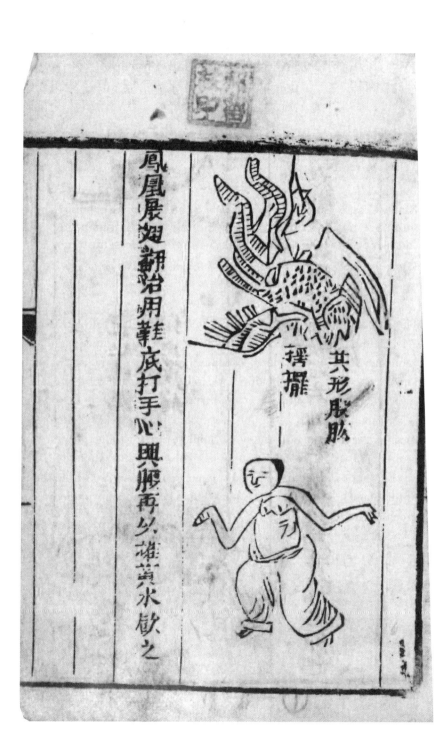

鳳凰展翅

其形最凶

搖擺

翎始用鞋底打手心與腿再以雄黃水歛之

P2. Black Gauze Cap Therapy
Wusha fan zhifa 烏紗翻治法

Nausea and Vomiting. Body Wracked with Pains.

Exin tupao. Hunshen tengtong.

惡心吐泡。渾身疼痛。

Black Gauze Cap Therapy. Use a needle and insert into the acupuncture points in the crook of the left and right arm, then smear the two points with realgar. That will relieve the symptoms.

Wusha fan zhifa. Yong zhen cipo zuoyou quchixue, zai yi xionghuang mo zhi, ji yu.

烏紗翻治法。用針刺破左右曲池穴，再以雄黄抹之，即愈。

The name of this therapy, *wusha* 烏紗, refers to a gauze hat black as a crow. Prior to the Manchu takeover of China in 1644, Han Chinese scholars and gentlemen kept their hair long. The hair was combed up and tied in a bun or topknot and it was common for many people to wear some kind of hat or hair covering. Scholars or officials often wore the black gauze hat referred to here.

Acupuncture is the use of needles inserted into the skin of the patient at specific points throughout the body. Studies suggest that acupuncture stimulates the release of the body's natural painkillers and affects areas in the brain involved in processing pain. It is recommended in a number of the therapies in this manual, sometimes alone but often in combination with decoctions of prepared herbs.

The specific acupuncture point called the Pool at the Bend (*quchixue* 曲池 穴) is on a key meridian of the internal system at the crease in the bend of the arm, so puncturing it with a needle should allow the normal flow of blood and *qi* 氣 within the body to resume. It is Acupuncture Point LI-11. For more discussion on this acupuncture point, see P38.

The phrase translated here as spit (*tupao* 吐泡) could also mean vomiting foam.

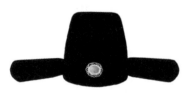

Traditional Chinese Horsehair Hat

惡心吐逆
渾身疼痛

烏紗翻治法用針刺破左右曲池穴再以雄黄抹之即愈

P3. Heavy Breathing Therapy
Chuiqi fan zhifang 吹氣翻治方

Presenting Symptoms: Heavy Breathing. Nervous and Unsettled.

Qi xing: Chuiqi. Xinhuang buning.

其形：吹氣。心荒不寧。

Heavy Breathing Therapy. Apply a needle at the Heavenly Gate. If this is not effective, apply the needle on both shoulders, and the front and back of the heart. That will bring relief.

Chuiqi fan zhifang. Yong zhen ci tianmen yi zhen. Ru bu hao, liang jian shang er zhen, qianhou xin ge yi zhen, ji yu.

吹氣翻治方。用針刺天門一針。如不好，兩肩上二針，前後心各一針，即愈。

The patient was clearly not calm. They might have been described as flustered (*xinhuang buning* 心荒不寧). By quickly looking at the patient and seeing the heavy breathing, it was clear to the medical practitioner that the major channels (*jingluo* 經絡) or meridians (*jingmai* 經脈) within the body were somehow clogged and not functioning smoothly. Note that Chinese traditional medicine uses both terms, channels and meridians, to refer to the flow of blood (*xue* 血) and energy (*qi* 氣) through the body, and in English both terms are often used indiscriminately. Western scientists accept the channels as physical conduits, but do not accept the idea of meridians as pure energy flows.

The points suggested where an acupuncture needle might be applied were among the most critical because they involved the head and the heart of the patient. Restoring smooth flow to that part of the body should have brought a sense of relaxation and calmness. The Heavenly Gate (*tianmen* 天門) is in the center of the forehead between the eyebrows, or perhaps a little higher where the "third eye" as seen in Daoist or Buddhist icons would be located. As an acupuncture point it is referred to as the Hall of Impressions (*yintang* 印堂). It is considered a non-channel accupuncture point, meaning that it does not lie on a meridian. It is sometimes listed as acupuncture point EM-2 or M-HN-3, dependng on the classification scheme used. This can treat frightening wind (*jingfeng* 驚風), high blood pressure (*gaoxueya* 高血壓), and frontal headache (*etoutong* 額頭痛). See Chan-Young Kwon and Boram Lee, "Acupuncture or Acupressure on *Yintang* (EX HN-3) for Anxiety: A Preliminary Review," *Medical Acupuncture* 30.2 (April 2018): 73–79, DOI: 10.1089/ acu2017.1268, PMCID: PMC5908420, PMID: 29682147. Also described in *Dictionary of Chinese Traditional Health* (*Zhongguo chuantong yangshengxue cidian* 中國傳統養生學辭典), ed. Zhuang Huafeng 莊華峰 and Fang Baiying 方百盈 (Nanning: Guangxi jiaoyu chubanshe, 1996), p. 727. The acupuncture points on the shoulders, shoulder well (*jianjing* 肩井), can help to relieve the feeling of shortness of breath. The acupuncture point is GB-21.

Note that the stamp on this page, and on most of the other pages in my copy of the manual, reads Hao Liugui 郝留桂, the name of the person who must once have owned this copy.

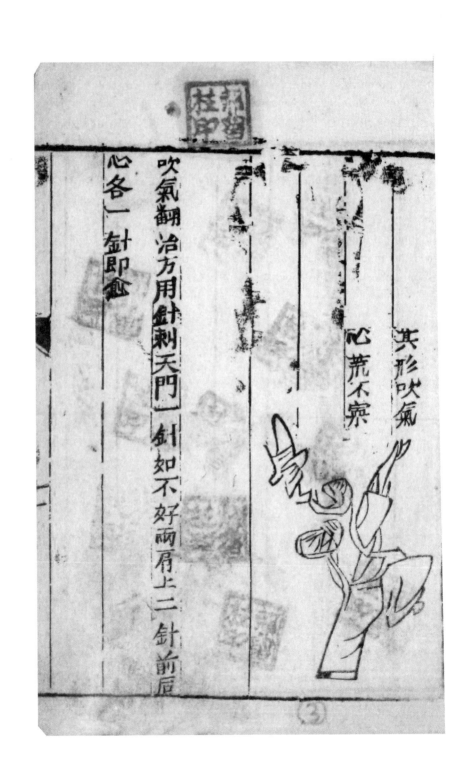

吹氣翻治方用針刺天門一針如不好兩肩上三針前辰

心各一針即愈

心荒不寧

其形吹氣

P4. Addled Brain Therapy
Hunnao fan zhi 混腦翻治

Bad Headache.

Naozi tengtong.

腦子疼痛。

Addled Brain Therapy. Take water used to boil black beans. Wet the sole of a [cotton] shoe and slap the top of the head to relieve the symptoms.

Hunnao fan zhi. Yong heidou zhu shui, xiedi jian zhi, da dingmen, ji yu.

混腦翻治。用黑豆煮水，鞋底湛之，打頂門，即愈。

Black beans, scientific name *glycine max*, contain the amino acid glycine which helps the body create a key detoxification enzyme called glutathione. Glutathione has been used to treat migraines. According to a study conducted by researchers at the University of Colombo in Sri Lanka, W. Pathirana et al., "Transcranial Route of Brain Targeted Delivery of Methadone in Oil," *Indian Journal of Pharmaceutical Science* 71.3 (May–June 2009): 264–269, it is possible "to deliver central nervous system drugs through the brain targeted transcranial route when applied on the scalp as oil solubilized dosage form. Systemic side effects of many common drugs could be overcome by the administration through the transcranial route since the drug targets the brain." Thus, it is possible that the slapping of the forehead might mean a slap on the top of the head in a way to rapidly get the medication into the scalp without troubling the patient by massaging the scalp.

A basic conception of the traditional Chinese approach to health was that the vital forces of the body needed to keep circulating within the body and an illness or uncomfortable feeling occurred when these forces were blocked from circulating. The purpose of slapping, striking, or hitting the patient was to knock out the blockage and allow the internal systems to continue their circulation. In the explanation of the therapy suggested, often the word used is *da* 打. Four of the medical recipes in this book recommend this action. The cloth shoe or sole soaked in water would be strong enough to jolt the patient and yet would not likely cause a bruise or break in the skin. A similar remedy is suggested in P8 below. The top of the head is called the Top Gate (*dingmen* 頂門). For comments on the *dingmen,* see P7 below.

Note that is no symbolic animal or insect assigned to this therapy.

脑子疼痛

混脑翻治用黑豆煮水鞋底熨之打顶门即愈

P5. Severe Itching Therapy
Naocuo fan zhifa 撓搓翻治法

Itching All Over the Body. Purple Boils Under the Tongue.

Hunshen cinao. She xia you ziding.

渾身刺撓。舌下有紫疔。

Severe Itching Therapy. Use a needle to pierce the purple boils under the tongue and let them bleed. That will relieve the symptoms.

Naocuo fan zhifa. Yong zhen cipo she xia ziding, chuxue, ji yu.

撓搓翻治法。用針刺破舌下紫疔，出血，即愈。

Purple boils refer to *ziding* 紫疔, painful pus-filled swellings of the skin and subcutaneous tissue caused by bacterial infection. This seems to have been a common complaint at the time this manual was prepared. In this manual I have translated the phrase as purple boils, sores, blisters, purple swellings, and pus-filled blisters. The word used to describe these eruptions in this manual is *ding* 疔 and they appear in much of the Chinese medical literature, sometimes modified as a black boil (*heiding* 黑疔) or purple-black (*zihei* 紫黑) boil. It is sometimes translated as a clove sore. In P41, I have translated the phrase (*ziqiding* 紫氣疔) as a purple blister. The *ding* 疔 could also be translated as a pustule, a pus-filled blister (*qiu* 丘), or pimple.

Medical therapies using the word *ding* 疔 in this manual are P5, P13, P16, P40, P41, P49, P50, P51, and P53. A descriptive guide for treatment is *Essential for Treating Pustules* (*Zhiding yaoshu* 治疔要書) (Shanghai: Hongda shanshuju, 1927), originally a woodblock cut in 1870. In P6, we encounter purple blisters (*zipao* 紫泡).

The *ding* 疔 and possible treatment with acupuncture are discussed in *Dictionary of Chinese Traditional Health* (*Zhongguo chuantong yangshengxue cidian* 中國傳統養生學辭典), ed. Zhuang Huafeng 莊華峰 and Fang Baiying 方百盈 (Nanning: Guangxi jiaoyu chubanshe, 1996), pp. 777–778. Also briefly in *Basic Chinese Medical Dictionary* (*Jianming Zhongyi zidian* 簡明中醫字典), ed. Yang Huasen 楊華森 et al. (Guiyang: Guizhou renmin chubanshe, 1985), p. 97.

This might be a description of a staph infection. Using a needle to drain boils under the tongue is now discouraged as it helps spread the infection. Current medical thinking reports that excessive body heat can cause the formation of painful, pus-filled heat boils on the body. Similarly, it can also cause the development of whitish, painful bumps under tongue. It appears the practitioner using this manual would quickly conclude that the swellings were caused by internal conditions within the body and were not a rash or other skin irritation. Letting the swellings bleed a bit would restore internal blood circulation and allow them to go away.

This therapy was translated as itching (*cinao* 刺撓), but the word also means scratching. No symbolic animal or insect was assigned to this therapy.

渾身刺撬

舌下有紫疔

撬撬翻治法用鍼刺破舌下紫疔出血即愈

P6. Disequilibrium Therapy
Bingyao fan zhifa 摒要翻治法

Presenting Symptoms: Stooped Over, the Mind Seems Docile, Fever, Vomiting, the Arms are Limp with Purple Blisters in the Armpits.

Qi xing: Juekua, yongxin, fashu, outu, gelao, zhi nei you zipao.

其形：蹶胯，雍心，發熟，嘔吐，胳捞，肢內有紫泡。

Disequilibrium Therapy. Use a needle to break the purple blisters and that will relieve the symptoms.

Bingyao fan zhifa. Yong zhen cipo zipao, ji yu.

摒要翻治法。用針刺破紫泡，即愈。

In classical Chinese medicine, the most crucial goal is to maintain an equilibrium within the body. When all of the systems are in place and the blood (*xue* 血) and *qi* 氣 flow smoothly, all is in harmony and the body functions. Here the presenting symptoms show the body is struggling against the imbalances within itself, even to the point of having the body stooped over and the arms limp. Crucial meridians connected with the heart (*xinzang* 心臟) and liver (*ganzang* 肝臟) run in the underarms and lower chest. Excessive underarm sweating, perhaps causing the blisters, is a sign of heat accumulation, which could be a product of poor diet, overwork, lack of sleep, or, more seriously, organ weakness. Puncturing the blood clots in the purple blisters is the first line of defense in restoring the system. The word used for this affliction, *bingyao fan* 摒要翻, means a therapy to adjust or get rid of the implied imbalance.

Like many of the entries in this book, the word purple (*zi* 紫) is used to describe the discolorations that occur either on or just underneath the skin. The color seems to refer to purple or dark red-black, noticeable discolorations indicating the accumulation of blood that is not free flowing. Gastrointestinal diseases would make sense for the fever, vomiting, limpness, etc., but not the boils. Stooping over fits the symptoms for opium overdose.

The skin swellings described here are sometimes translated as pustules or bloated eruptions in this manual. The term appears in P6, P13, P39, and P40.

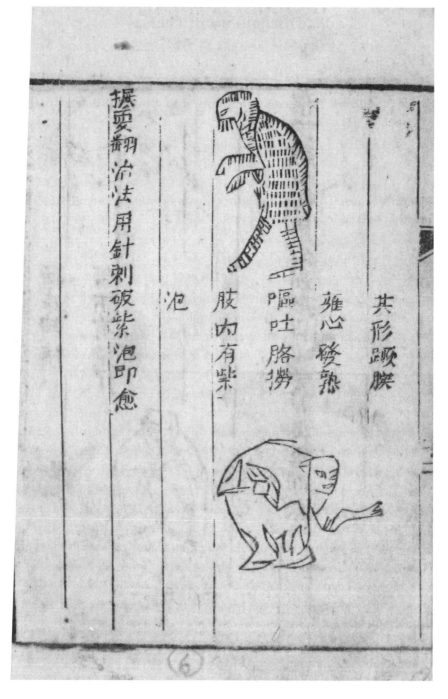

其形踞躟

驚心發熱

嘔吐膈勞

肢內有紫

泡

撮要翻治法用針剌破紫泡即愈

P7. Long Snake Therapy
Changchong fan zhifa 長蟲翻治法

On the Ground, Rolling on the Floor, Stomach Pains. Flatulence.

Jiudi dagun. Duzhang.

就地打滾。肚脹。

Long Snake Therapy. Into the navel insert three needles, then two needles will go into the *dingmen*, then in the soles of the left and right feet, one in each foot. Wipe the area with tobacco tar to affect relief.

Changchong fan zhifa. Xian tiao duqi san zhen, ci tiao dingmen liang zhen, zuoyou jiaoxin ge yi zhen. Yong yanyou shi zhi, ji yu.

長蟲翻治法。先挑肚臍三針，次挑頂門二針，左右腳心各一針。用煙油拭之，即愈。

The *dingmen* 頂門 refers to the crown or the top of the head, or to the high forehead. See *A Chinese-English Dictionary* (*Han-Ying cidian* 漢英詞典) (Beijing: Foreign Language Teaching and Research Press, 2010), p. 311. A phrase used in the Republican period (1912–1949) for the high forehead was Gate to the Brain (*naomenzi* 腦門子). See *Concise English-Chinese Dictionary*, ed. Shau Wing Chan (Stanford, CA: Stanford University Press, 1946), p. 106. The dictionary word used today for this part of the body is *etou* 額頭 or *emen* 額門. See *New Age Chinese-English Dictionary* (*Xinshidai Han-Ying da cidian* 新時代漢英大詞典) (Beijing: The Commercial Press, 2007), p. 393. The *dingmen* is mentioned in this manual in P4, P7, P8, and P33.

The acupuncture point in the soles of the feet would probably be KI-1, the Bubbling Well (*yongquan* 湧泉). In this manual the arch in the sole of the foot (*jiaoxin* 腳心) is mentioned in P7 and P38. The foot (*zu* 足) is mentioned in P21.

After the isolation of nicotine from tobacco leaves in 1828, the medical world in the West became more mistrustful of tobacco as a general treatment and aware that the plant contained a dangerous alkaloid. Nicotine began to be used alone and more effort was made to measure doses. For example, a preparation of nicotine salicylate as a 0.1% salve replaced an infusion of leaf tobacco boiled in water as a treatment for scabies. Tobacco, however, was still seen as a strong ointment to clean away noxious irritants. Tobacco smoke was sometimes still recommended for conditions as varied as strychnine poisoning, constipation, strangulated hernia, tetanus, hydrophobia, and worms. See Anne Charlton, "Medicinal Uses of Tobacco in History," *Journal of the Royal Society of Medicine* 97.6 (June 2004): 292–296.

Until the mid-1800s tobacco was seen as a medical herb with positive therapeutic qualities. "[T]here undoubtedly was a real belief in the medicinal efficacy of tobacco, especially within the context of the fifteenth and sixteenth century notions of health and disease. For example, certain diseases were seen as a disturbance in the balance of four qualities: hot, dry, cold, and wet. Catarrh (the common cold), particularly prevalent in the northern countries, was believed to be due to excess of cold and wet, so that applications of hot and dry tobacco smoke was seen as beneficial." See Juan R. Sanchez-Ramosa, "The Rise and Fall of Tobacco as a Botanical Medicine," *Journal of Herbal Medicine* 22 (August 2020), DOI: 10.1016/j.hermed.2020.100374.

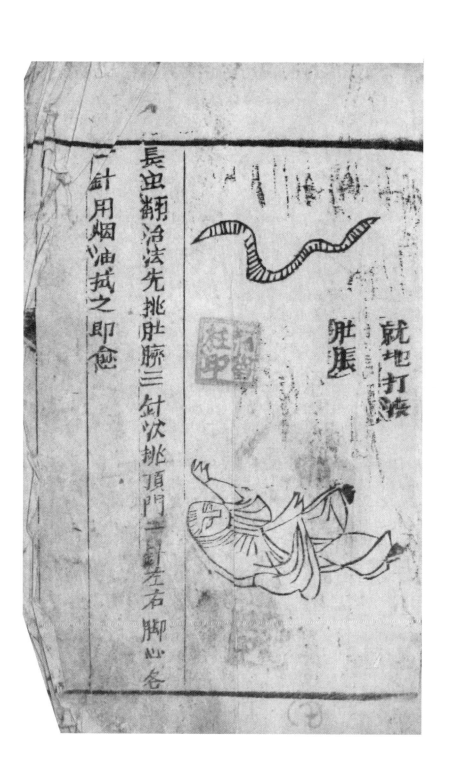

長虫顙治法先挑肚臍三剳次挑頂門一剳左右脚心各一剳用烟油拭之即愈

就地打滾

肚脹

P8. Being Dumb [Unable to Speak] Therapy
Eba fan zhifa 噁叭翻治法

Unable to Stand or Speak.

Zhaodi, bu nen yanyu.

着地，不能言語。

Being Dumb [Unable to Speak] Therapy. Take the sole of a [cotton] shoe that has been wetted with cold water and strike the top of the head. Have a woman dip her hands in cold water and pat the head.

Eba fan zhifa. Yong xiedi jian liangshui, da dingmen. Nüren fenfa, yong shou jian liangshui, pai zhi.

噁叭翻治法。用鞋底湛涼水，打頂門。女人分髮，用手湛涼水，拍之。

See the explanation for P4 above, that the purpose of hitting or slapping the patient was intended to knock away the blockage that was preventing the fluids of the body from continuing to flow. Having the woman part her hair means the center of the scalp would be exposed because the hair would be parted in the middle of the scalp.

However, medical advice tells us that a woman's hand are actually cooler than the hands of a male. See Han Kim et al., "Cold Hands, Warm Heart," *Lancet Letters* 351, Issue 9114 (May 16, 1998): 1492, https://www.thelancet.com/journals/lancet/article/PIIS0140-6736%2805%2978875-9/fulltext, accessed April 11, 2021. For example, if the medical condition was like a stroke or epilepsy, a heat (*yang* 陽) situation with seizures that are clenched and spastic, then the coolness of a female's hands were cool (*yin* 陰), and that would have a soothing effect on the patient's condition.

Most of the afflictions in this manual could affect either males or females, but the illustrations made for this collection almost always depict males. At the end of this collection are several unillustrated medical recipes; those could also affect males, but some are more specific to females or children. Is that why they were unillustrated and placed at the end of this collection? Chinese historical medical text did illustrste women and children, but only in a small number of instances.

著地不能

官語

噎以酒治法用鞋底泥涼水打頂門灸人分髮用手焦涼

衣抱之

P9. Toad Therapy
Hama fan zhifa 蛤蟆翻治法

This Affliction: Bloated Stomach.

Qi zheng: duzhang.

其症：肚脹。

Toad Therapy. Into the area of the belly button [navel] insert seven acupuncture needles, and insert three acupuncture needles into the area of the lower abdomen. That will offer relief.

Hama fan zhifa. Duqi yuanwei tiao qi zhen, xiaodu tiao san zhen, ji yu.

蛤蟆翻治法。肚臍圓圍挑七針，小肚挑三針，即愈。

In Chinese traditional medicine, excessive gas was seen as being caused by a deficiency of *qi* 氣 in the spleen (*pi* 脾); in other words, a weak digestive system not working properly. The presenting symptoms all seem to indicate this as the most obvious cause of the symptoms. This is a case where the application of the acupuncture needles all take place in the immediately affected area of the body. This is of note because often with acupuncture the needles are placed somewhere along an affected channel (*jingluo* 經絡) in an area that might be removed from the area of the body where the pain or discoloration, etc. is located.

This swelling in Chinese is called water swelling (*shuizhong* 水腫), in Western medicine often termed edema. This is an abnormal accumulation of water in the body caused by impairment of the transformative action of *qi* 氣 in the lung (*fei* 肺), spleen, and kidney (*shen* 腎). Another term used in Western medicine is dyspepsia. One cause of the swelling could be a peptic ulcer. Most commonly one finds cases of functional dyspepsia, which are swellings caused by a problem like indigestion and results in stomach aches, a feeling of fullness, or an uncomfortable bloating after meals. The use of acupuncture needles to relieve the discomfort of functional dyspepsia is common today in Chinese medicine. Comments on this problem can be found in "Acupuncture for Stomach Pain & Bloating?" site of Andrew Hubbard, September 2, 2019, https://drandrewnd.com/acupuncture-for-functional-dyspepsia/ (accessed May 18, 2021).

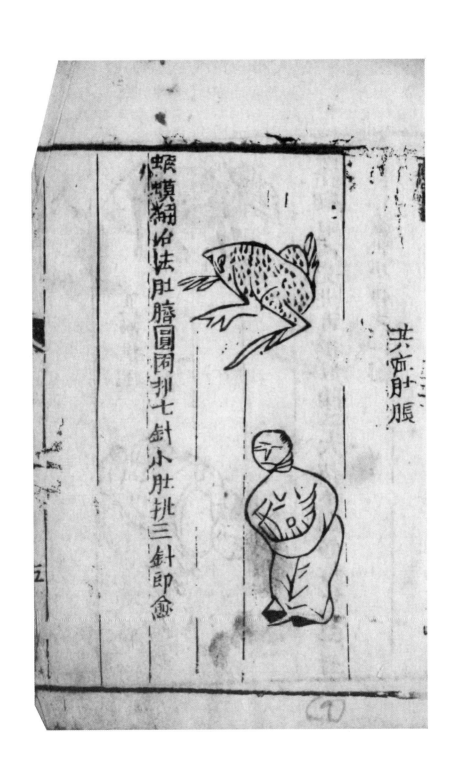

蝦蟆翻治法肚臍圓閞挑七針小肚挑三針即愈

共血肚脹

P10. Sow Disease Therapy
Muzhu fan zhifa 母豬翻治法

Presenting Symptom: Rooting on the Ground.

Qi xing: Gongdi.

其形：拱地。

Sow Disease Therapy. First insert a needle at the back of the tongue, then except for the two thumbs, apply one needle to each of all the other fingers. Then wet the tongue with swill [liquid pig feed], that will relieve the symptoms.

Muzhu fan zhifa. Xian tiao shegen, hou chu er dazhi bu zhen, yuzhi ge zhen yi zhen. Zai yi zhushi chishui guan zhi, ji yu.

母豬翻治法。先挑舌根，後除二大指不針，餘指各針一針。再以豬食池水灌之，即愈。

The tongue was considered a crucial indicator of the condition of the internal organs. The tongue was felt to have a special connection to the heart, as expressed in the phrase "the heart opens to the tongue" (*xin kaiqiao yu she* 心開竅於舌). This implies that disturbances of the heart are invariably reflected in the tongue. The tongue itself can change color, or it can be affected by dark blood stasis (blood that is not circulating) speckles. Chinese doctors today still feel that an examination of the tongue provides important information about the patterns of vital circulation or blockage within the body. Many of the treatments presented in this manual begin with examining and treating the tongue.

Pig swill was composed of scraps from uneaten meals and could be strong in nutrients. In most Chinese households pig feed consisted of scraps of uneaten food, usually in a soft or liquid form. Depending on the family's diet, this could be composed of bean cake, rice chaff, corn, and eggshells. This could have the effect, for pigs and humans, of increasing digestion, clearing scourge, and vanquishing toxins. Research on the nutritional value of pig swill is reported in: Cao Guowen 曹國文, "Research into Chinese Herbal Medicine and the Modern Uses of Raising Pigs" (*Zhongcaoyao zai jindai yangzhuye zhong de yingyong yu yanjiu* 中草藥在近代養豬業中的應用與研究), *Szechuan Animal Husbandry and Veterinary Medicine* (*Sichuan xumu shouyi* 四川畜牧獸醫) 28.11 (2001): 31–32.

其形拱地

母猪翻治法先挑舌根后除二大指不針餘指俱針一齒

兩以猪食池水灌之即愈

P11. Body Numbness Therapy
Mashazhang zhifang 麻殺脹治方

This Affliction: The Entire Body Is Numb [tingling sensation].

Qi zheng: Bianshen muma.

其症：遍身木麻。

Body Numbness Therapy. Use a plant stock [that is hard; don't peel off the skin] soaked in water to strike the thighs and forearms. Then look for bluish color [skin discoloration bruises], which will relieve the symptoms.

Mashazhang zhifang. Yong dai pi magan jian liangshui, da gugongqiong. Jian qing, ji yu.

麻殺脹治方。用帶皮麻扞，湛涼水，打股肱穹。見青，即愈。

Blood stasis, being clogged up and not moving normally, can be revealed by some discoloration of the skin in body extremities. In classical Chinese medicine, numbness often stems from deficiencies in the liver (*ganzang* 肝臟), kidneys (*shen* 腎), and spleen (*pi* 脾). The pathogenic factors could be caused by wind (*feng* 風), cold (*han* 寒), and dampness (*shi* 濕). Striking the limbs with a wet or damp cloth, or in this case the lower part of a firm or hard plant stock, was meant to help restore smooth blood flow to the limbs. The phrase in this prescription, *dai pi magan* 帶皮麻扞, means to use the plant stock with the skin still on it. Similar therapies of striking the patient as a therapy are seen in the examples above on P4 and P8. When the striking produces discoloration in the skin, it could be taken as a sign that the clogged blood has been dislodged and is rising to the surface of the skin, a good indication that normal blood flow is resuming.

Numbness was felt to be caused by a combination of the pathogens (*xie* 邪) of wind, cold, and dampness. They could cause localized pain in the muscles and joints, restricted physical movement, and numbness. It was necessary to free the internal network vessels, thus the need to strike the limbs to a point of allowing the blood to flow, as would be seen by the developing bruises. The word *xie* 邪 means "evil," but here it is translated as the medical term "pathogen."

No symbolic animal or insect was assigned to this therapy.

其症遍身

木麻

麻殺脹治方用帝皮麻挼湛涼水打股肚窩見青即愈

P12. Mole Cricket Therapy
Lougu fan zhifa 螻蛄翻治法

Presenting Symptoms: Swelling of the Breasts. Painful Lumps on the Breasts. Tingling or Rough Feeling.

Qi zheng: Ru liang pang si lougu. Chuang xing ciyang, shi nanren.

其症：乳兩旁似螻蛄。瘡形刺癢，是難忍。

Mole Cricket Therapy. Stir-fry wheat bran with salt and vinegar and rub it [on the affected area].

Lougu fan zhifa. Yong yan cu, chao fuzi, shi zhi.

螻蛄翻治法。用鹽醋，炒麩子，拭之。

The instruction to stir-fry (*chao* 炒) was one method of reducing herbal ingredients to a powder or ash. Described as "Tossing materials in a heated wok; the most common form of heat processing. Stir-frying in the context of medicinal processing, in contrast to cooking, means dry frying: oil should never be used unless specifically stated." This explanation continues in Nigel Wiseman and Andy Ellis, *Fundamentals of Chinese Medicine* (Brookline, MA: Paradigm Publications, 1995), p. 491. Other therapies recommending stir-frying in this manual are P45, P61b, and P61e.

Swelling (distention, *ju* 疽) of the breasts can be caused by menstrual irregularities or the condition of constriction-blood disharmony. In this case the practitioner wants to cure the discomfort, which is producing a tingling or rough feeling, perhaps as if a cricket was crawling over the sensitive breasts. The advice is to rub the prepared ointment on the affected area and not have recourse to any invasive measures.

In this case the affliction is named after the itching sensation it causes. Correcting this condition employs the practice of harmonization (*hefa* 和法) to rectify the *qi* 氣 that vitalizes and propels the body, and to harmonize it with the construction *qi* (*yingqi* 營氣) that also helps to animate the body. The construction *qi* forms the blood and flows with it, helping to nourish the entire body. It is said to be distributed among the bowels (*changzi* 腸子) and thus can enter the blood vessels. The phrase used for harmonization is "rectify the *qi* and harmonize the construction" (*liqi heying* 理氣和營).

This is an example, as the illustration seems to show, of a female malady.

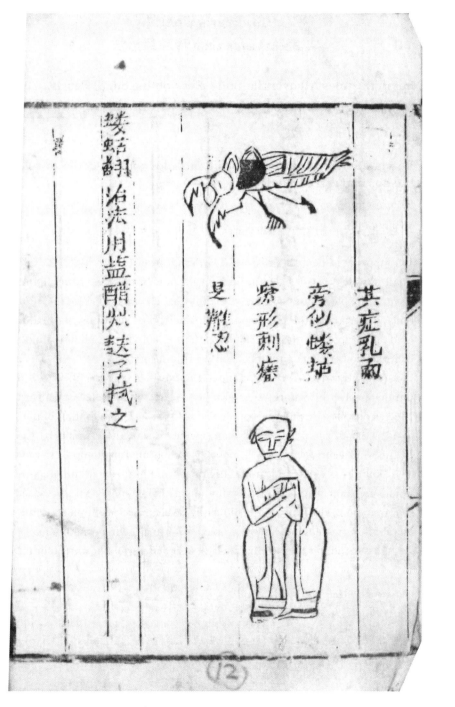

其症乳兩

旁作悸怵

瘆形刺癢

是難忍

蟆蛤翻治法用塩醋㷔送子拭之

P13. Pearls Therapy
Zhenzhu fan zhifa 珍珠翻治法

Small Pustules All over the Body, Resembling Small Pearls.

Shen shang qipao, si zhenzhu yang.

身上起泡，似珍珠樣。

Pearls Therapy. Just prick all the pustules with a needle to release the pus and effect relief.

Zhenzhu fan zhifa. Yong zhen, bian zhen jian xue, ji yu.

珍珠翻治法。用針，遍針見血，即愈。

This appears to be a skin disease. The "small pearls" (*zhenzhu* 珍珠) refer to small pustules (*pao* 泡) that are filled with pus. In this case restricted movement of the blood and *qi* 氣 along the internal channels (*jingluo* 經絡) of the body were causing the condition. Removing the clogged pus that had gathered and erupted on the skin would open the channels and allow the blood to continue flowing. The pus is probably whitish in color.

In my translation of this manual, the pustules that are filled with deep red or purplish blood are referred to as *ding* 疔, which I have usually translated as pustules. Pustules or papules (*qiu* 丘) are a slight elevation of the skin filled with pus or blood. In Chinese medical terms these would be caused by the wind evil (*fengxie* 風邪), possibly complicated by damp heat (*shire* 濕熱). Skin diseases can appear and disappear and in this case the practitioner would not want to confuse the eruptions as being simply a rash caused by skin irritation. The skin rash could easily be a surface phenomena, while the blood-filled pustules indicated a problem involving the internal organs.

This is another therapy that was not assigned a symbolic animal or insect.

身上起泡

似珍珠樣

珍珠翻治法用針逼肘見血即愈

P14. Lamb Disease Therapy
Yanggao fan zhifa 羊羔翻治法

The Voice Is Like the Bleating of a Sheep, with Foaming at the Mouth.

Sheng ru yangming, kou zhong tumo.

聲如羊鳴，口中吐沫。

Lamb Disease Therapy. Mix a concoction of realgar, white cicada, and ginger juice in cold water and drink it down.

Yanggao fan zhifa. Yong xionghuang, baifan, chan, jiangzhi he liangshui, song xia.

羊羔翻治法。用雄黃、白礬、蟬、薑汁和涼水，送下。

Ginger was one of the popular items in early trade within Asia and along the Maritime Silk Road. Oil taken from the ginger plant, the "ginger juice" (*jiangzhi* 薑汁) mentioned here, is well-known as a medicine to prevent nausea and vomiting. It generally has no known side effects. Ginger juice has beneficial effects on the tongue, which may have a white "furry" look. Molting from a cicada (*chan* 蟬) is used as an anti-allergy medication which helps support the nose, sinus, and respiratory system. It can be used to clear the lungs and loss of voice. The yellow rice wine (*huangjiu* 黃酒) was made from glutinous rice and wheat. It was perhaps the most common alcoholic drink among rural people in north and northeast China.

Realgar (*xionghuang* 雄黃), which can be translated as "masculine yellow," is toxic and can be poisonous. It was considered able to ward off evil, just as it could ward off snakes and rodents if sprinkled around the house. It was used carefully in small amounts in classical Chinese medicine after having been burnt to ashes and then added to yellow rice wine, water, or tea. Several other medical recipes in this manual prescribe the use of realgar. From the frequency of it being prescribed, we can assume it was considered to be an easily available and acceptable drink among a majority of the people.

Note that this is one of the few medical recipes recommending the use of cold water as the liquid decoction.

聲如羊鳴

口中吐沫

平羔翻治法用雄黃白礬蟬姜汁和家水送下

P15. Horse Therapy
Macu zhifa 馬粗治法

Presenting Symptoms: Heavy Breathing, Limbs Weak and Chilled.

Qi zheng: hangchuan, sizhi ju liang.

其症：吭喘，四肢俱涼。

Horse Therapy. Take the mastication of a horse and add some yellow [realgar] and yellow rice wine. Drink it down to effect a cure.

Macu zhifa. Yong majiaohuan, shang shenghuang. He huangjiu song xia, ji yu.

馬粗治法。用馬嚼環，上生黃。和黃酒送下，即愈。

The phrase indicates using the mastication of a horse (*majiaohuan* 馬嚼環). This could mean to take from the horses' mouth horsefeed that it has been chewing and that had gathered on the harness bit in its mouth. Horsefeed was often a collection of a family's garbage, but not including meat or bones, usually composed of grains which the horse would chew into a fine mixture. Possibly it was the mixture of nutrients from the grains mixed with the horse's saliva that would be benificial.

The Chinese doctor might deduce that this person is suffering from a situation where the normal flow of blood and vital fluid in the body has been stopped. According to a Chinese doctor friend consulted during my translation of this manual, the practitioner recommending this prescription might have prescribed salvia (*danshen* 丹參), an herb in the mint family. It can affect the chemistry of the brain to produce mild opiate-like symptoms. Medically it was considered a blood-quickening, stasis-transforming agent, meaning it would break the log-jam preventing the smooth flow of blood and vital forces to make the flows more rapid, to relieve the patient's condition.

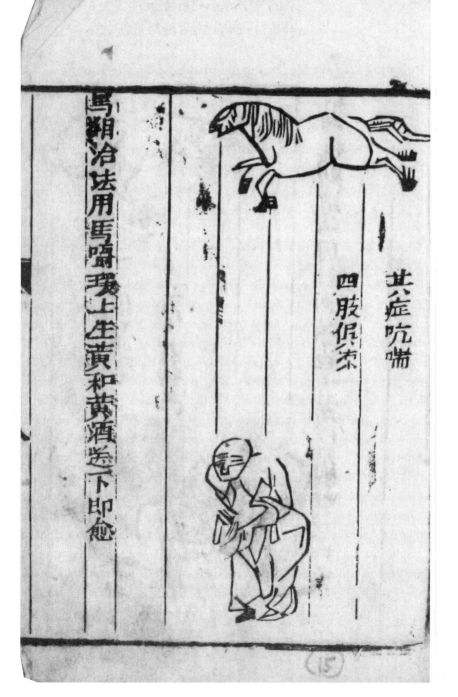

馬瘵冷法用馬噴遽上生黃和黃酒送下即愈

其症咆喘

四肢俱冷

(15)

P16. Donkey Therapy
Shequlü fan zhifa 蛇曲驢翻治法

Pulsating Like the Heart. Purple Blister Under the Tongue.

Chuxin zhanzhan. She xia you ziding.

傗心戰戰。舌下有紫疔。

Donkey Therapy. Use a needle to puncture the purple sore under the tongue and apply a little tobacco tar. That will bring relief.

Shequlü fan zhifa. Yong zhen cipo she xia ziding, yanyou dian zhi, ji yu.

蛇曲驢翻治法。用針刺破舌下紫疔，煙油點之，即愈。

This animal is actually not a donkey, nor is it a snake. It seems to refer to a donkey which is curved like a snake. People got sick like this, with hands and legs in the air. Howls of pain like a donkey but the body bent as a snake. The donkey as pictured in the illustrations usually accompanying this therapy had an elongated body somewhat resembling a supple snake, hence the phrase used to name this addiction: "slithering snake donkey" (*shequlü* 蛇曲驢)?

On the rapid heartbeat, a common image in the Western mind is that of the donkey being a beast of burden. Slow, perhaps, but strong and often given work that seemed to task its strength, like carrying heavy loads or pulling large wagons. Those burdens imposed on the donkey might have caused it to exert all its power, resulting in a rapid heartbeat similar to the rapid heartbeat exhibited by the patient who approached the practitioner.

There can be several reasons for a rapid heartbeat. Among them are stress, anxiety, or some stumulant like caffeine. In this case the doctor only knew that it was important to bring the heartbeat down to normal by getting the constricted blood to flow smoothly by puncturing the sore under the tongue (*she xia ziding* 舌下紫疔), and then applying tobacco tar as a soothing medication, which would have been a common prescription in 1860s China.

蛇門驢雜治法用針刺破舌下紫疔烟油點之即愈

舌下有紫疔

僧心戰人

P17. Turtle Therapy
Gui fan zhifa 龜翻治法

With This Ailment, the Head Falls Forward Causing Distress, with Dark Veins at the Temples.

Qi zheng: Shentou, wanyao xinteng, liang bin you zijin.

其症：伸頭，彎腰心疼，兩鬢有紫筋。

Turtle Therapy. Needle the purple veins to allow flow, and apply realgar to affect relief.

Gui fan zhifa. Yong zhen tiaopo zi, yi shi guoyu, you shanghuang, dian zhi, ji yu.

龜翻治法。用針挑破紫，以使過魚，又上黃，點之，即愈。

In this affliction the person has a bent back and seems to be continually bowing, as if a humble person is meeting a higher status person. In naming this affliction, it must have been thought the condition was as if the patient were carrying a heavy object on their back, causing them to be bent forward as they moved. This does not seem to refer to a hunchback (*yulou* 傴僂) although the afflicted person referred to here finds it impossible to assume a straight posture, which is one of the definitions of a hunchback condition.

The thearpy assumes that the discolored tendons are restricting the flow of blood, which is caused by the neck straining forward. Sometimes a bent posture, which would be a dysfunctioning of the spinal muscles, has a neurological cause; the basal ganglia nuclei of the cerebral cortex are malfunctioning with the result that the body positioning causes a bent posture to occur. The symptoms of the discolored neck veins seen by the Chinese practitioner could indicate this was the case and applying some acupuncture therapy would bring about the most rapid relief.

Note that the label of this affliction appears to use the word *fan* 翻 to mean disease or medical condition. Is the illustration of a male or a female?

其症伸頭
彎腰心疼
兩脅有紫
筋

用針挑破紫絲以使過了血又上黃点之即愈

P18. Ox Head Therapy
Niutou fan zhifa 牛頭翻治法

Symptom: Continual Noise in the Ear Like an Ox Bellowing.

Qi zheng: Sheng ru niuming.

其症：聲如牛鳴。

Ox Head Therapy. Using realgar, grind up cicada molting and black beans into a powder. Drink with cold water.

Niutou fan zhifa. Yong xionghuang, chantui, heidou wei mo. He liangshui song xia.

牛頭翻治法。用雄黃、蟬退、黑豆為末。和涼水送下。

This appears to be a case of extreme tinnitus. The herbal recipe suggests using the discarded skin molting of a cicada (*chantui* 蟬 蛻). Cicadas were considered to counter the effects of wind-caused diseases. This implies that the practitioner who prepared this therapy assumed the cause was wind (*feng* 風). In classical Chinese medicine, this pathogen would have been called an evil wind (*xiefeng* 邪風).

The word for cicada molting is written as *chantui* 蟬退. Notice the second character is pronounced the same as the correct character, however the similar-sounding but mistaken character was written. Selecting a wrong character that sounded the same as the intended character was a common mistake made especially by people with a limited formal education.

Black beans (*heidou* 黑豆) were black soybeans which had many positive effects on health, including relieving the uncomfortable effects of headaches and nausea. It is possible that some of the noise in the ear from tinnitus is caused by the flow of blood through the neck and head. The black soybeans could thin the blood to a degree where it flowed more easily which decreased the noise in the ears. Placing these in the context of medical prescriptions in pre-modern China is in Andrew Schonebaum, *Novel Medicine: Healing, Literature, and Popular Knowledge in Early Modern China* (Seattle: University of Washington Press, 2016), pp. 149–150.

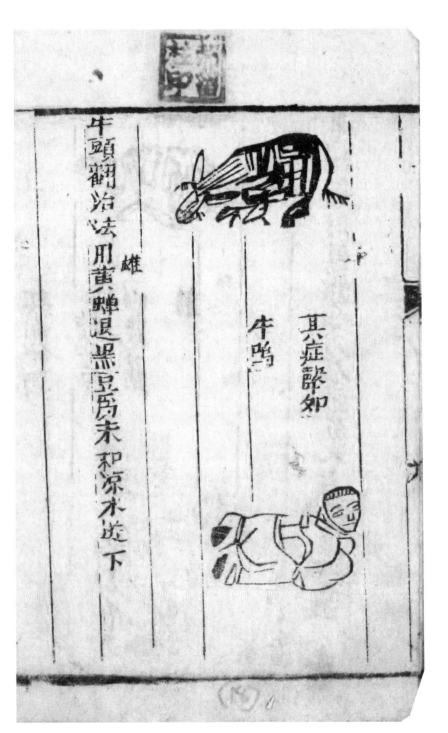

牛頭瘟治法　用黄蟬退黑豆為末和涼水送下

雄

牛鳴

其症醉如

P19. Mule Affliction Therapy
Luozi fan zhifa 騾子翻治方

Ears Feel Cool, Legs Are Stretched Out, Cannot Bend.

Er liang, shentui, bu neng zhang.

耳涼，伸腿，不能張。

Mule Affliction Therapy. Take the sediment from a trough used by anmials and burn it to a powder. Add it to yellow rice wine, and pour in some vinegar [to be drunk]. That will bring relief.

Luozi fan zhifa. Yong caodi yuliao wei mo. He huangjiu, chencu guanzhi, ji yu.

騾子翻治方。用槽底餘料為末。和黃酒、陳醋灌之，即愈。

This seems to be a case of stiff joints and a temporary paralysis of the legs. The ears feel cold, so something is not flowing to the extremities. The sediment at the bottom of a trough used by animals would likely be composed of grains and fodder, if not the cores of apples or berries and other fruits, left-over grains, etc. These foods that had been discarded by humans and mixed in with animal fodder would be filled with vitamins and protein that would restore vigor and strengthen the the vital systems within the body (*huoqi* 活氣) of the human in distress.

We have seen the same process at work in P15 explained above. Making use of every possible source of nutrition was among the practices of Chinese farmers who often had to live using their own resources, taking what was at hand and could be beneficial.

耳涼仲腿

不能張

騾子剛始方用胡椒餘料為末和黃酒陳醋灌之即愈

P20. Bean Worm Therapy
Douchong fan zhifa 豆蟲翻治法

Shaking the Head and Wagging the Tail.

Yaotou baiwei.

搖頭擺尾。

Bean Worm Tharapy. Insert one accupuncture needle at the Heavenly Gate. Take the rust from a used hoe and apply it three times [repeatedly]. That will bring relief.

Douchong fan zhifa. Yong zhen ci tianmen yi zhen, yi shi guo chuban shang shenghuang, lian dian san ci, ji yu.

豆蟲翻治法。用針刺天門一針，以使過鋤板上生黃，連點三次，即愈。

The Heavenly Gate (*tianmen* 天門) is considered to be between the eyebrows or slightly higher in the center of the forehead, where the "third eye" seen on some deities would be located. As explained in P3 above, as an acupuncture point it is referred to as the Hall of Impressions (*yintang* 印堂), which is considered a non-channel accupuncture point, meaning that it does not lie on a meridian. It is sometimes listed as acupuncture point EM-2 or M-HN-3, dependng on the classification scheme used.

In Chinese classical thinking, metal (*jin* 金) is one of the key elements of life. Using scrapings of rust from a farmer's hoe might have been a way to take the restorative elements of metal and increase them in the system of the distressed patient. Among the mineral elements of metal that have nutritional significance for human health are chromium, cobalt, copper, iodine, iron, manganese, nickel, selenium, and zinc. Such elements can be toxic when levels exceed a certain threshold but otherwise are considered beneficial to the body.

Essential mineral deficiencies (*xu* 虛) may be present in patients with chronic illness. For example, persons suffering from iron deficiency exhibit anemia and its corresponding symptoms of fatigue, pallor, and dizziness.

In this case the practitioner was seeing involuntary movements from the afflicted person. Involuntary movement is called dystonia. This condition involves sustained involuntary muscle contractions with twisting, repetitive movements. Dystonia may affect the entire body or only certain parts. Other examples of involuntary movement, such as P1 above where the arms flap (*gugong yaobai* 股肱搖擺), or in P40 below, were sometimes encountered.

搖頭擺尾

豆虫翻治法用針刺天門一針以使為鋤板上生黃連点

三久即愈

P21. Binding Up Therapy
Chanmian fan zhifa 纏綿翻治法

Appears Deranged. Stomach Pains, Headache. Has an Unnatural Posture and Appearance. Mind Seems at a Loss. Bloodshot Eyes.

Xinshazi fang, yi ju yu ci. Duzhang, touteng, xinfan, qianhouxin you qing, huang, ziyan.

心殺子方，亦具於此。肚脹，頭疼，心翻，前後心有青、黃、紫眼。

Binding Up Therapy. Using an acupuncture needle to prick the blue, yellow, purple discolored areas, and apply vinegar. If the person seems unresponsive and immobile, then a person without responses is one whose mind has gone. Use an acupuncture needle placed in the hands, feet, or wrist. Decoct boiled salt, that will bring relief.

Chanmian fan zhifa. Yong zhen tiaopo qing, huang, zi deng yan, yi cu cha zhi. Ruo hunshen muma wu dian zhe, shi xinshazi ye. Yong zhen jiang shou, zu, wan tiaopo. Chaoyan jianfu, ji yu.

纏綿翻治法。用針挑破青、黃、紫等眼，以醋搽之。若渾身木麻無點者，是心殺子也。用針將手、足、腕挑破。炒鹽煎服，即愈。

Because of using too much ink during the printing process, the characters naming this therapy were smudged and are difficult to read in my copy of the manual. The first character of the therapy, *chan* 纏, means to bind up or to bandage. The second character is *mian* 綿, often used to mean cotton wadding. In my woodblock copy it apppears to be *cai* 綵, meaning blood. This is now the commonly used meaning of the character, but according to some dictionaries it means "blood from a wound." See *New Age Chinese-English Dictionary* (*Xinshidai Han-Ying da cidian* 新時代漢英大詞典) (Beijing. The Commercial Press, 2007), p. 139.

The presenting symptoms which the doctor saw indicated some rather serious condition had taken hold. Though the causes were not clear, the need was to bring about emergency relief as quickly as possible. One could assume that there were times when a patient was encountered with these indications of an extreme condition. It might have been the result of a fight or an accident but the afflicted person was not able at that juncture to assist by giving details. They may have been in a near comatose state.

No symbolic animal or insect was assigned to this therapy. It might have been difficult to designate which creature to assign.

心殺子方　肚張頭疼

亦具於此　心翻前后

心有青黄

紫眼

稠糊冷法用刀桃破青黄紫等眼以醋捺之若渾身木

麻無點者是心殺子也用刀將手足腕挑破炒盐煎服即

愈

P22. Fish Therapy
Yu fan zhifang 魚翻治方

Presenting Symptoms: Nausea. Stomach Hurts As If from Drinking Too Much Water.

Qi zheng: Exin. Duo yinshui, du zhong tengzhang.

其症：惡心。多飲水，肚中疼脹。

Fish Therapy. Take a fishnet and burn it. Treat the patient by combining the ashes with yellow rice wine. After some sweating, the symptoms will be relieved.

Yu fan zhifang. Yong shi yu yuwang shaohui, huangjiu tiaofu. Chuhan, ji yu.

魚翻治方。用使遇魚網燒灰，黃酒調服。出汗，即愈。

This could be a case of indigestion, but in this case it is described as overhydration: too much liquid. Drinking too much water which is not eliminated from the body can cause water levels to build up. This dilutes important substances in the blood. Nausea is a common symptom, along with a bloated feeling. Were Chinese in the Qing period prone to drinking too much tea?

This therapy suggests a fishnet which most likely has a lot of the detritus of fish on it which would then be transferred to the patient through drinking the decoction. This can be considered a quick and inexpensive way to obtain the chemicals that fish possess. Fish contain high-quality protein, iodine, and various vitamins and minerals. Fatty varieties have omega-3 fatty acids and vitamin D. A fish in the diet is linked to reduced mental decline in older adults. Presumably the remains of the cooked fish would also act as a diuretic to relieve the nausea and stomach pain.

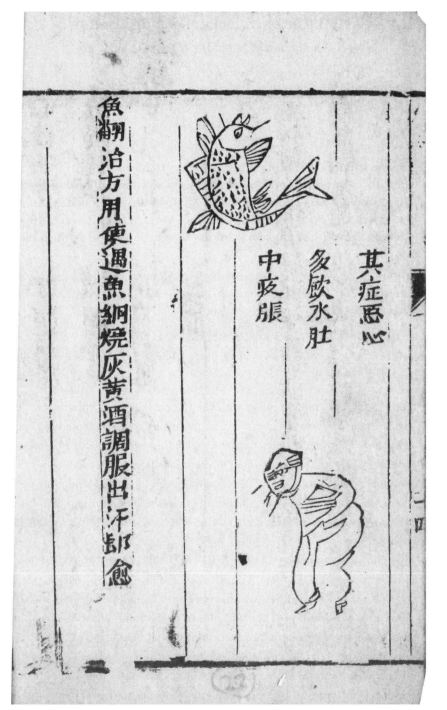

其症惡心

多欲水肚

中疰脹

魚翻 治方用使遇魚網燒灰黃酒調服出汗卽愈

P23. Uncontrollable Bleeding Therapy
Xueliu bu zhi fan zhifa 血流不止翻治法

Uncontrollable Bleeding.

Xueliu bu zhi.

血流不止。

Uncontrollable Bleeding Therapy. Use tendons from a living person. To stop the blood flow, bind them up, bake them on a stove. Drink them with yellow rice wine. This should bring relief. No matter where the body bleeds you cannot stop it, that is the nature of this condition. Use human tendons, fingernails, and to stop bleeding, human hair.

Xueliu bu zhi fan zhifa. Yong huoren jin, shi xueyu chan jia. Lu wei ximo, huangjiu song xia, ji yu. Fan yi shen bulun hechu, xueliu bu zhi, ji cizheng ye. Huoren jin, ren zhijia ye. Xueyu, ren toufa ye.

血流不止翻治法。用活人筋，使血餘纏佳。爐為細末，黃酒送下，即愈。凡一身不論何處，血流不止，即此症也。活人筋，人指甲也。血餘，人頭髮也。

Could this be a symptom of hemophilia? Uncontrollable or continuous bleeding were serious presenting symptoms. According to the accepted analysis of classical Chinese medicine, continuous bleeding had several likely causes: *qi* deficiency (*qixu* 氣虛) was making blood vessels fragile and unable to contain blood; excessive heat (*duore* 多熱) had damaged blood vessels and made the blood move in improper ways; blood stasis (*xuezhi* 血滯) was causing obstructions in blood vessels resulting in the blood outflowing from its normal pathways.

The idea is to use human fingernails and human hair (*crinis carbonisatus*), bind them up and bake them. The ash would be injested with yellow rice wine.

Medical doctors tell us that fingernails and toenails are composed largely of keratin (*jiaodanbai* 角蛋白), a hardened protein that is also found in hair. In this case the medical prescription calls for both human nails and hair to be heated and then drunk with wine. Experiments have shown that recombinant keratins can enhance fibrin clot formation at the site of injury and decrease the bleeding time and blood loss. This was reported in Tingwang Guo,

Wenfeng Li, Ju Wang, Tiantian Luo, Deshuai Lou, Bochu Wang, and Shilei Hao, "Recombinant Human Hair Keratin Proteins for Halting Bleeding," *Artificial Cells, Nanomedicine, and Biotechnology: An International Journal,* 46:sup2 (April 2018): 456–461, DOI: 10.1080/21691401.2018.1459633. Another recipe to stop bleeding using human fingernails and/or toenails is in Bao Xiangao 鮑相璈, *Raising the Dead and Returning Life: Emergency Medicine of the Qing Dynasty* (*Qisi huisheng* 起死回生), trans. Lorraine Wilcox (Portland, OR: Chinese Medical Database, 2012), p. 124.

No symbolic animal or insect was assigned to this therapy.

血流不止

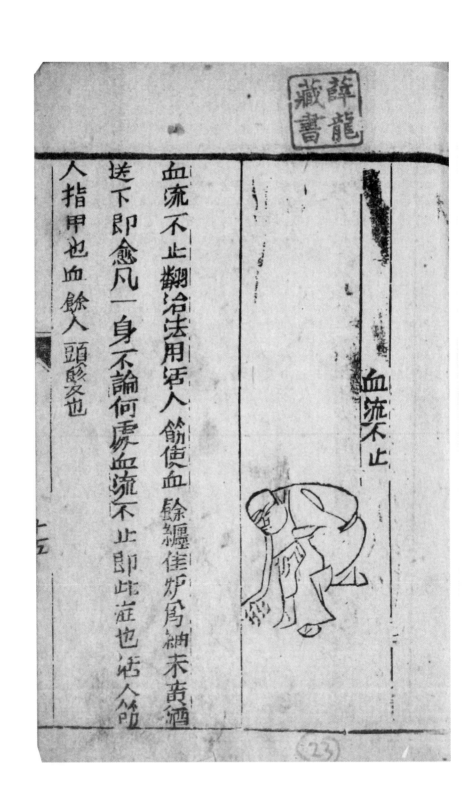

血流不止翻治法用活人觔使血餘纏住炉為細末黃酒

送下即愈凡一身不論何處血流不止即此症也活人觔

人指甲也血餘人頭髮是也

P24. Deer Disease Therapy
Lu fan zhifang 鹿翻治方

Spitting Blood. Purple Spots on the Body. Person with Syphilis.

Koutu xuemo. Shenshang fazi. Ban si you meihua zhe.

口吐血沫。身上發紫。斑似有梅花者。

Deer Disease Therapy. Use a needle to prick the purple spots. Mix ground deer antler into a gelatinous state, and drink it with yellow rice wine. That will being relief.

Lu fan zhifang. Yi zhen cipo bandian. Ci yong lujiao jiao, he huangjiu song xia, ji yu.

鹿翻治方。以針刺破斑點。次用鹿角膠，和黃酒送下，即愈。

The comment that "the spots look like syphilis" (*ban siyou meihua zhe* 斑似有梅花者) was the usual way of referring to someone with this affliction; those with veneral disease were described as someone with "plum flowers" (*meihua* 梅花). This was in reference to the purple sores that could spring up all over the body. These sores are usually (but not always) firm, round, and painless. Symptoms of secondary syphilis include skin rash, swollen lymph nodes, and fever. To have the rash and be spitting blood, it appears this person has a case of syphilis that is advancing in the body.

In recent studies a panel of Chinese researchers concluded that "deer antler base possess immunomodulatory, anti-cancer, anti-fatigue, anti-osteo-porosis, anti-inflammatory, analgesic, anti-bacterial, anti-viral, anti-stress, anti-oxidant, hypoglycemic, hematopoietic modulatory activities and the therapeutic effect on mammary hyperplasia." See "Deer Antler Base as a Traditional Chinese Medicine: A Review of Its Traditional Uses, Chemistry and Pharmacology," *Journal of Ethnopharmacology* 145.2 (January 30, 2013): 403–415. Could this be the reasoning behind labeling it "Deer Disease Therapy"?

Deer antlers were among the herbs and animal parts that were extensively used in traditional Chinese medicine and which became commercially produced. The story of how this happened is described in Liz P. Y. Chee, *Mao's Bestiary: Medicinal Animals and Modern China* (Durham, NC: Duke University Press, 2021).

口吐血沫

身上發紫

班似有梅

花者

麋翻治方以針刺破班點以用鹿角膠和黃酒送下即愈

P25. Camel Disease Therapy
Luotuo fan zhifa 駱駝翻治法

Foaming at the Mouth. Purple Boil Behind the Ears.

Kou fa baimo. Er hou you ziding.

口發白沫。耳後有紫疔。

Camel Disease Therapy. Use a needle to break open the boil. Burn dried ox dung, mix with a fragrant oil, and daub it on the area.

Luotuo fan zhifa. Yong zhen cipo ziding. Yi gan niufen shaohui, xiangyou he cha.

駱駝翻治法。用針刺破紫疔。以乾牛糞燒灰，香油和搽。

In this case, the practitioner must have suspected that a restricted flow of blood caused the blood to back up, visible in the protruding boil. The remedy was to prepare a salve and apply it on the opened boil. Cow dung has been used in many cultures to make bricks for building structures. When caked and dried it has been used as fuel for heating, and as an agricultural fertilizer. In some parts of the developing world it is collected and used to produce biogas to generate electricity and heat.

A text from early Ireland propsed using the dung of various animals for its medicinal effects. See Ranke De Vries, "A Short Tract on Medicinal Uses for Animal Dung," *North American Journal of Celtic Studies* 3.2 (2019): 111–136.

It is claimed by some that ox dung cures skin ailments from eczema to gangrene. Those people believe that the medicinal properties of herbs eaten by cows and oxen when they are out in the fields remain in the cow dung. Moreover, cow dung contains a substance similar to penicillin, which has a disinfecting effect and reduces the bacteria that cause diseases.

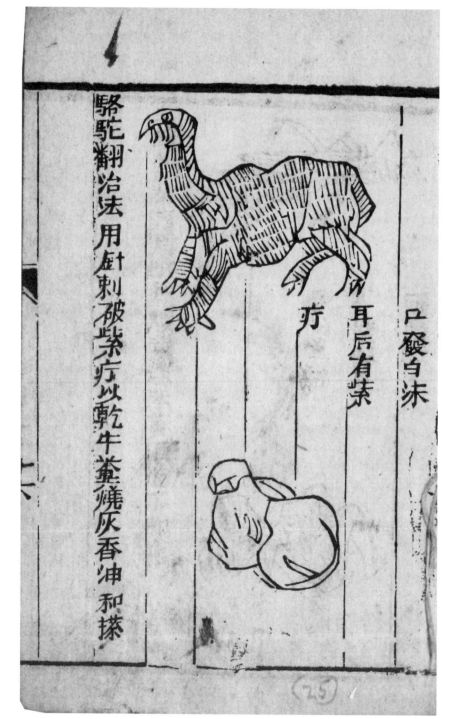

駱駝翻治法用針刺破紫疔以乾牛糞燒灰香油和搽

尸發白沫

耳后有紫

疔

P26. Grasshopper Therapy
Jila fan zhifang 蟣蠟翻治方

Legs Trembling. Unable to Stretch. Nausea. Mental Condition.

Liangtui zhanzhan. Bu neng shuzhan. Exin. Xinfan.

兩腿戰戰。不能舒展。惡心。心翻。

Grasshopper Therapy. Roast a grasshopper to ashes. Add this to yellow rice wine and drink it down. That will bring relief.

Jila fan zhifang. Yong jila duanhuang wei mo, huangjiu song xia, ji yu.

蟣蠟翻治方。用蟣蠟煅黃為末，黃酒送下，即愈。

Similar to muscle cramps, spasms occur when a muscle involuntary and forcibly contracts and cannot relax. This is a common occurrence and can affect any muscle. Massage to relax the muscle seems an immediate response, but in modern medicine various chemical compounds can also be used. Americans often turn to Tylenol. In sympathetic medicine, the affliction is defined as related to a certain animal or action, as in this case of "Grasshopper affliction."

In this text the word for roasting is written "heat up" (*duan* 煅). This word is also seen in P29 below. Another word used for roasting is *wei* 煨. Warming or heating the ingredients for a medicinal recipe will draw out unwanted oils or irritants and reduce their toxicity. In many medicial recipes there are a number of ingredients. They can be heated by putting them in wet paper, or coating them in flour and water paste then placing them on embers until the wrapping becomes burnt and black. Other methods of heating include putting them on the side of the fire, or in an oven, or into a wok (*guo* 鍋). See Nigel Wiesman and Andrew Ellis, *Fundamentals of Chinese Medicine* (Brookline, MA: Paradigm Publications, 1995), p. 489.

Grasshoppers are classified as *Orthoptera*. They are eaten as a snack in East Asia. They are also used in Asian medicines in China, India, and Korea, as well as in Mexico and Latin America. They provide treatments against rheumatism, warts, urine retention, and other maladies. Known anticancer agents pancratistatin and narciclasine, and an additional derivative, ungeremine, have been isolated from grasshoppers. Several of these compounds were "further tested against murine lymphocytic leukemia cells and a variety of human tumor cell lines and as expected all were active against the cell lines with narciclasine being the most potent on each cell line." See Lauren Seabrooks and Longqin Hua, "Insects: An Underrepresented Resource for the Discovery of Biologically Active Natural Products," *Acta Pharmaceutica Sinica B* 7.4 (July 2017): 409–426.

Note the phrase used here in the presenting symptoms section of the description, mental condition (*xinfan* 心 翻), is an indication that the word *fan* 翻 was used to mean a disease.

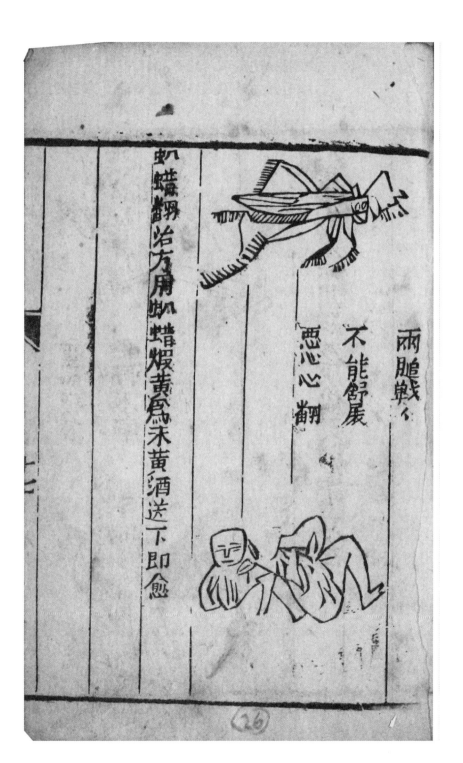

兩腿戰

不能舒展

惡心嘔

蚱蟷翻治方用蚱蟷煨黃爲末黃酒送下即愈

P27. Spinning Wheel Therapy
Fangchezi fan zhifa 紡車子翻治法

Nausea and Dizziness. Unable to Relax or Sleep.

Exin, touhun. Zuowo buning.

惡心，頭昏。坐臥不寧。

Spinning Wheel Therapy. Take thread from the spinning wheel. Burn it to ash, and combine it with yellow rice wine. Drink to effect a cure.

Fangchezi fan zhifa. Yong xian chao hui. Wei huangjiu song xia, li yu.

紡車子翻治法。用絃炒灰。為黃酒送下，立愈。

Cotton thread as used for spinning wheels was long and continuous and moved smoothly through the loom. Such is the quality of good sleep, so symbolically the type of cure hoped for was to silently flow through the loom of sleep. Spinning wheels were common in homes in pre-modern China as well as in many other countries, since making clothes and repairing them was a typical and recurring aspect of home life. The women of the family were always making clothing, scarves, towels, shoes, handbags—anything that could be made with cloth.

Cotton is used to alleviate nausea, fever, headache, diarrhea, dysentery, nerve pain, and bleeding. See Mary A. Egbuta, Shane McIntosh, Daniel L. E. Waters, Tony Vancov, and Lei Liu, "Biological Importance of Cotton By-Products Relative to Chemical Constituents of the Cotton Plant," *Molecules* 22.1 (January 2017): 93. These authors write that "Cotton is described as a medicinal plant because of the chemical compounds that have been isolated from it. A number of compounds found in cotton play pharmacological roles in nature including anti-microbial, anti-inflammatory, cytotoxic, anti-cancer, and contraceptive roles in both humans and animals. Monoterpenes such as myrcene, pinene, camphene, limonene, and sabinene isolated from cotton possess anti-microbial, anti-inflammatory, anti-cancer, anti-oxidant, and gastro-protective properties."

Some medical practitioners in old China seem to have felt that drinking too much poorly made spirits like rice wine could also bring on all of the symptoms listed above. For example see Bao Xiangao 鮑相璈, *Raising the Dead and Returning Life: Emergency Medicine of the Qing Dynasty* (*Qisi huisheng* 起死回 生), trans. Lorraine Wilcox (Portland, OR: Chinese Medical Database, 2012), p. 80.

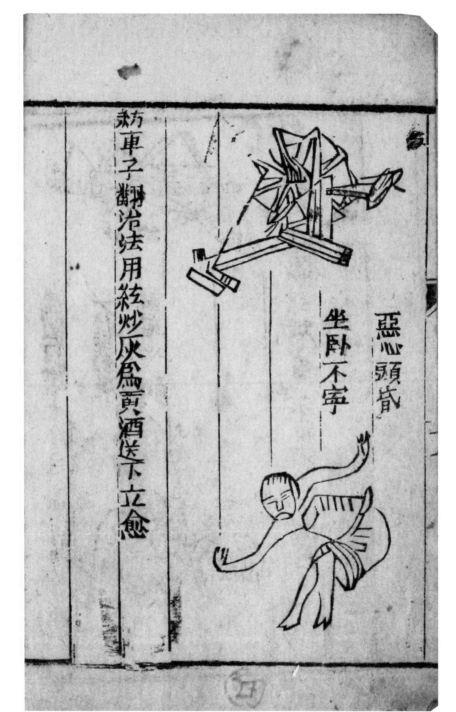

惡心頭疼

坐臥不寧

紡車子翻治法用絃炒灰爲頭酒送下立愈

P28. Earth Dragon [Snake] Therapy
Dilong fan zhifa 地龍翻治法

Rolling Around on the Ground. Pain in the Small Intestine. Flatulence.

Jiudi dagun. Xiaochang tengtong. Duzhang.

就地打滾。小腸疼痛。肚脹。

Earth Dragon [Snake] Therapy. Take some fat used to grease the spinning wheel and burn it. Combine it with rice wine and drink down. That will effect a cure.

Dilong fan zhifa. Yong younianzi shaohui. Huangjiu song xia, li yu.

地龍翻治法。用油捻子燒灰。黃酒送下，立愈。

The snake is called the earth dragon (*dilong* 地龍) because actual dragons can fly in the sky or go under the sea, while the snake stays on the earth. We assume that the grease used on spinning wheels in the farmer's homes was animal fat. "Animal fats occupy a unique position of utilization in the pharmacopeia of Chinese traditional medicine. Animal fats used in Chinese folk remedies are those found in the periphery far away from the marrow." Although the animal fats used include a large variety of animals, from domestic to wild types, "they share a common indication of 'replenishing' for the malnutrited or debilitated. Another common use is for skin conditions like various types of injuries and infections." See Ping Chung Leung, "Use of Animal Fats in Traditional Chinese Medicine," in N. Bhattacharya and P. Stubblefield (eds.), *Regenerative Medicine* (London: Springer, 2015), pp. 73–76.

To relieve the pain caused by gas or indigestion, the lubricating grease used to keep home spinning wheels in continuous use was easily available. The ashes of the burnt oil, mixed with rice wine, was the cure prescribed here. Perhaps like the popular pre-modern and not pleasant-tasting laxative castor oil?

就地打滚

小肠疼痛

肚胀

地龍翻治法用油捻子燒灰黃酒送下立愈

P29. Nine Doses for Distress Therapy
Jiu zhong xinteng zhifa 九種心疼治法

Distress.

Xinteng.

心疼。

Nine Doses for Distress Therapy. Take sap from the *huai* tree, burn it to ash. Add vinegar and form into a pill as large as a green bean. Drink nine pills each time with water that has been boiled.

Jiu zhong xinteng zhifa. Yong huairou duanhuang wei mo, chencu wei wan, ru lüdou da. Meifu jiu wan, baishui song xia.

九種心疼治法。用槐肉煅黃為末，陳醋為丸，如綠豆大。每服九丸，白水送下。

For the medical practitioner to encounter a patient who feels distressed, upset, or tormented seems to have been a common condition for most of the afflictions described in this manual. Modern Chinese medical dictionaries describe this psychological state as a "troubled mind" (*kunao* 苦惱).

The *huai* 槐 tree (*sophora japonica*), a large tree which grows in North China, is medically credited with cooling the blood, cooling the liver fire which causes red eyes and dizziness. It is known in English as the scholar tree or the pagoda tree. It is a favorite plant for use in classical Chinese medicine and its parts have many beneficial uses. For several recipes using the flowers of the *huai* tree in decoctions to calm agitated patients, see Bao Xiangao 鮑相璈, *Raising the Dead and Returning Life: Emergency Medicine of the Qing Dynasty (Qisi huisheng* 起死回生), trans. Lorraine Wilcox (Portland, OR: Chinese Medical Database, 2012), pp. 151–155.

"Modern pharmacological studies and clinical studies demonstrated that these chemical constituents [of the scholar tree] possess wide reaching pharmacological actions like antioxidant, anticancer, antiasthmatic, antineoplastic, antimicrobial, antiviral, antidote, antipyretic, cardiotonic, antiinflammatory, diuretic and in the treatment of skin diseases like eczema, colitis and psoriasis." See Murali Krishna Panthati, K. N. V. Rao, S. Sandhya, and David Banjii, "A Review on Phytochemical, Ethnomedical and Pharmacological Studies on

Genus *Sophora,* Fabaceae" *Revista Brasileira de Farmacognosia* 22.5 (September/ October 2012): 1145–1154.

In the recipe above, the manual has the word *duan* 煅 which means to change something into an ashy powder by heat, to calcify. Throughout the manual this action is usually written as *shao* 燒, to burn. The character *duan* 煅 is occasionally used in this manual, as in P26 above.

No animal or symbolic illustration was assigned in my manual for this affliction.

心疼

九種心疼治法用槐肉煨黃為末陳醋為丸如綠豆大

每服九丸白水送下

P30. Insect Therapy
Chong fan zhifang 蟲翻治方

First a Swollen Head, Then Swollen Legs, Finally a Swollen Back.

Xian zhong tou, ci zhong tui, hou zhong yao.

先腫頭，次腫腿，後腫腰。

Insect Therapy. Take mulberry leaves, boil in water and wash the entire body. Then burn the vines of a Chinese trumpet creeper [*tecoma grandiflora*], add that to the water of the boiled mulberry leaves and drink down to effect a cure.

Chong fan zhifang. Yong sangye shao shui, bianshen xi zhi. Zai yi tiaocao shao-hui, he sangyeshui yin zhi, li yu.

蟲翻治方。用桑葉燒水，遍身洗之。再以苕草燒灰，和桑葉水飲之，立愈。

The presenting symptoms are bloated parts of the body, so whatever the internal probem, portions of the skin are swollen and probably uncomfortable. Washing the body with the medicinal lotion would be a good first step. This is followed by mixing the boiled vines with the medicinal water from the boiled mulberry leaves (*sangyeshui* 桑葉水) and drinking it down.

Mulberry trees have been cultivated in China for centuries. The bark of the tree is used to make a sturdy paper much admired by calligraphers and painters in East Asia. In addition, the mulberry leaves are used to feed the worms that produce silk cocoons, and silk was one of the important items produced in China and then traded all along the famous Silk Road (*Sichou zhi lu* 絲綢之路) as early as the second century BCE. The effects of mulberry leaves to relieve swelling has been studied by scientists. One example is Enkyo Park et al., "Anti-Inflammatory Activity of Mulberry Leaf Extract Through Inhibition of NF-κB," *Journal of Functional Foods* 5.1 (January 2013): 178–186. Among the findings of Park and their team of researchers was that "Mulberry leaf has been traditionally used to treat chronic diseases such as diabetes and cancer. The effect and mechanism of mulberry leaf extract (MLE) in LPS-induced activation of macrophage was investigated by the levels of production of proinflammatory mediators and cytokines, and their transcriptions. . . .

[R]esults suggest that MLE can be used as an anti-inflammatory agent to inhibit NF-κB-mediated inflammatory response." A similar investigation is in Hyun Hwa Lim et al., "Anti-Inflammatory and Antiobesity Effects of Mulberry Leaf and Fruit Extract on High Fat Diet-Induced Obesity," *National Library of Medicine* 238.10 (October 2013): 1160–1169, DOI: 10.1177/1535370213498982.

This is another case where no symbolic animal or insect was assigned as a label for this condition.

先腫頭

次腫腿

后腫腰

虫翻治用桑葉燒水遍身洗之再以莨草燒灰和采莧

水散之立愈

P31. Constricted Eyesight [Sparrow's Eyes] Therapy
Quemu fan zhifang 雀目翻治方

Presenting Symptom: As If at Dusk, Cannot See Clearly.

Qi zheng: Ru huanghun shi, bu neng jianwu.

其症：如黃昏時，不能見物。

Constricted Eyesight [Sparrow's Eyes] Therapy. Take roots of the alfalfa plant, boil them and drink them with water.

Quemu fan zhifang. Yong muxugen shao shui, yin zhi.

雀目翻治方。用苜蓿根燒水，飲之。

The word used for this therapy, sparrow's eyes (*quemu* 雀目), refers to the idea that sparrows have a very poor eyesight in the evening or at night. Sparrows are active in daylight so do not need night vision. Scientists say the makeup of the cone cells in their retina gives them poor night vision.

Alfalfa is is a leafy green vegetable. It is a general observation of doctors that leafy green plants contain compounds that will benefit good eyesight. These contain nutrients like omega-3 fatty acids, lutein, zinc, and vitamins C and E that can help ward off age-related vision problems like macular degeneration and cataracts.

Among the plants recommended to help promote good eyesight are green leafy vegetables such as spinach, kale, and collards. One of these plants is lucerne, also called alfalfa (*muxu* 苜蓿). It is cultivated as an important forage crop in many countries around the world, where it is most commonly used for grazing, hay, and silage, as well as a green manure and cover crop. It was known to the Chinese, especially in North China where horses and mules were common in rural areas. The Chinese doctor might also have assumed the patient's poor eyesight was a temporary problem that developed rapidly, possibly caused by high blood sugar levels. High blood sugar causes the lens of the eye to swell, which changes the ability to see. To correct this kind of blurred vision, one needs to get blood sugar back into the target range.

In place of the word *shao* 燒 (to burn down or to boil) used here, some printed versions of these medical recipes used the word *jian* 煎 which means to simmer in water to decoct medicinal herbs.

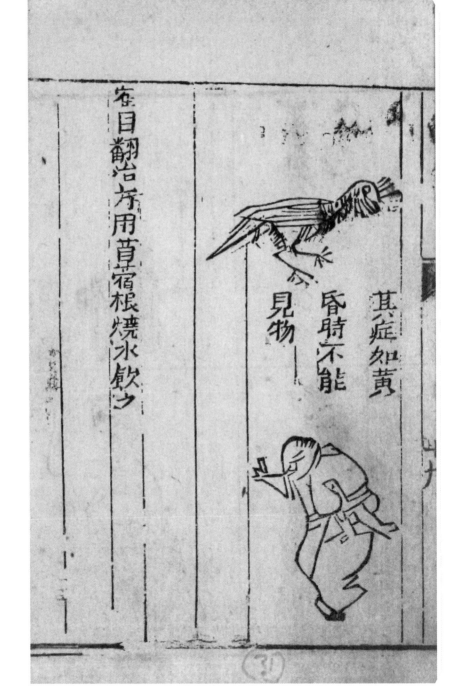

其症如黃

昏時不能
見物

安目翻治疗用苜蓿根燒水飲之

P32. Bloated Stomach Therapy
Yongxin fan 壅心翻

Bloated Stomach.

Duzhang yongxin.

肚脹壅心。

Bloated Stomach Therapy. If the condition has been persistent, it will be difficult to cure. Quickly use five portions of realgar and drink it with cold water. After one or two doses the ache in the belly and the condition will be relieved.

Yongxin fan. Shi jiu nan zhi. Jiyong xionghuang wu fen, he liangshui song xia. Yi er shi fuxiang, ji yu.

壅心翻。時久難治。急用雄黃五分，和涼水送下。一二時腹響，即愈。

Concerning the phrase *yi er shi fuxiang* 一二時腹響 (one or two doses [goes into the belly]), the meaning of the phrase can be translated as above, which conforms to the 1916 versions of these medicinal therapies I have seen. As written in my 1860s version, the word time (*shi* 時) would be close to the vernacular way of expressing the phrase.

As we we have seen in this manual beginning with P1, realgar (*xionghuang* 雄黃) is made from a toxic powder that can be considered a poison, so it is diluted in water or rice wine when ingested as a medicine. In this case the stomach bloating needs to be relieved, so five *fen* 分 of realgar (about 0.08 ounce) should be dissolved in cold water and drunk down by the patient.

Pure realgar by itself has low toxicity. Moreover, its poor solubility hampers its absorption by the gastrointestinal tract. Its absorption would be further weakened by having it mixed with cold water as specified in this prescription. In most cases the Chinese practitioner would prescribe that realgar be mixed with heated water or (warmed) rice wine, which would increase its absorption into the body. In this case the practitioner did not want to poison the patient, but only to take advantage of the curative power of the realgar to bring down the bloating (*chen* 膩).

Note that no animal or insect was assigned as a label for this affliction.

肚腹甕心

甕心翻時久難治急用雄黃五分和涼水送下一二時腹

响即愈

P33. Struggling with Discomfort
Dingshazhang fa 頂殺脹法

Headache and Heartburn. Vomiting and Diarrhea.

Naoteng tongxin. Shangtu xiaxie.

腦疼痛心。上吐下瀉。

Struggling with Discomfort. Take cold water and slap it on the forehead to bring relief.

Dingshazhang fa. Yong liangshui, da dingmen, ji yu.

頂殺脹法。用涼水打頂門，即愈。

In the anlaysis of classical Chinese medicine, nausea, vomiting, and diarrhea indicate too much dampness (*shi* 濕 or *yin* 陰) in the stomach. To dispel the cold and warm up the body, one could eat gently warming foods such as ginger, millet, oats, turnips, or carrots.

However, in an effort to very quickly remove the condition from the patient, this prescription calls for jolting the patient out of their discomfort by striking the forehead with cold water. For comments on the term *dingmen* 頂門 that refers to the crown of the head or the high forehead, see P7 above. If water is prescribed as part of a decoction to be injested, it is usually served warm or hot, but in this case it is put on the head as a stimulant for external use and cold water will have a better effect. From the practitioner's point of view, a rapid cure with elimination of the stasis would always bring thanks and praise from the afflicted.

No symbolic animal or insect is used to label this condition.

頂殺脹法用涼水打頂門即愈

腦疼痛心

上吐下瀉

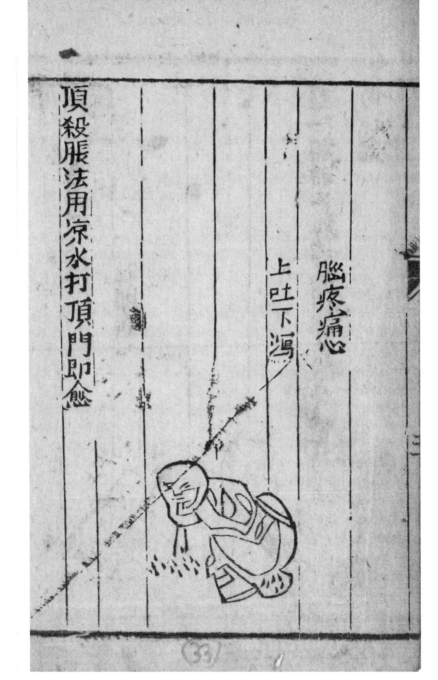

P34. Horse Monkey Therapy
Mahou fan zhifa 馬猴翻治法

Headache. Nausea. Vomiting.

Touteng. Exin. Outu.

頭疼。惡心。嘔吐。

Horse Monkey Therapy. Use the ends of a leather riding whip and burn them to ashes. Drink with rice wine.

Mahou fan zhifa. Yong pibian shao, shaohuang wei mo. Huangjiu song xia.

馬猴翻治法。用皮鞭梢，燒黃為末。黃酒送下。

What is the Horse Monkey (*mahou* 馬猴)? It seems the Chinese internet has a number of answers to this question. For example, in the northeastern Jiaodong and Weihai region of Shandong province 山東省膠東威海, the term "horse monkey" refers to the cicada (*chan* 蟬). The slough (*chantui* 蟬蛻) or empty skeleton of the cicada is employed in classical Chinese medicine. It affects the lung (*fei* 肺) and the liver (*ganzang* 肝臟). It relieves the symptoms of spasm, skin rashes, eye and throat discomfort. If we look at the illustration on this page of the manual, we see it could be a cicada slough.

But there is another credible explanation for a horse monkey. It is a large simian named the mandrill in the monkey family that has a prominent snout giving its face somewhat of a resemblance to a horse. It can reach a shoulder height of 20 inches (50.8 cm). Its home is in equatorial Africa, but it was known to the Chinese. A reference to it appeared in the novel *Dream of the Red Chamber* (*Hongloumeng* 紅樓夢) first published in China in a woodblock edition in 1791. In Chapter 28 (*ershiba hui* 二十八回) one of the women in the mansion reported: "She was distressed when a large horse monkey bolted out of the embroidery room!" (*Nüer chou, xiufang cuanchu ge damahou* 女兒愁，繡房竄出個大馬猴). See Cao Xueqin 曹雪芹 (1710–1765), *Dream of the Red Chamber* (Cheng Yi Edition) (*Hongloumeng [Cheng Yi ben]* 紅樓夢 [程乙本]) (Beijing: Beijing Tushuguan chubanshe, 2001), Vol. 2, p. 380, line 5; Zhou Ruchang 周汝昌 and Chao Jizhou 晁繼周, eds., *Dream of the Red Chamber Dictionary* (*Hongloumeng cidian* 紅樓夢辭典) (Guangzhou: Guangdong renmin chubanshe, 1987).

But why is this image in a literati novel? It seems the image of a large monkey was used to frighten children and get them listen to the adults. It was called the commander of all the ghosts (*yiqie guishen de tongling* 一切鬼神的統 領) and the demon of the spirit (*jingshen emo* 精神惡魔). The child should be obedient, listen to their parents, eat when told to, and go to sleep when the adults say. If children disobey, the horse monkey will come and take them away. In this regard, the horse monkey was an ogre used to frighten people. It appears that was how the image was used in the *Dream of the Red Chamber*. If the artist's supposed rendering of the horse monkey in my manual resembles anything, it is a formless and vaguely menacing apparition. Does the illustration of the patient represent the female in the novel who was startled by the horse monkey? If so, it is one of the few times a female patient is drawn in the manual.

In this case the presenting symptoms could be referring to dysphoria, which can include the symptoms listed above along with a sense of discomfort, distress, or unease. Could the use of the ends of a horse whip have some symbolic meaning? After all, a whip is used to tame an animal, so using it may help calm the patients.

What about burning the ends of a horse whip? Perhaps the use of the whip ends is symbolic of striking the patient, a remedy suggested in several other therapies in this manual. Is it going too far to say that using the ends of the leather whip which had struck the animal hides was a way to take advantage of the nutrients that might have gathered on the animal bodies? It is doubtful the practitioner in the 1860s had this concept in mind.

On the internet I found a plant called the Horse Monkey Beak (*mahou zhuazi* 馬猴爪子). It can grow on roofs between the tiles. It can be used medically as a detoxant (*jiedu* 解毒) and to stop bleeding (*zhixue* 止血).

The ideas associated with this animal go on and on. This is one of the more enigmatic recipes in the manual.

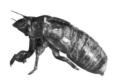

Cicada Skeleton
(image by USDA, CC BY 2.0)

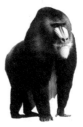

Horse Monkey

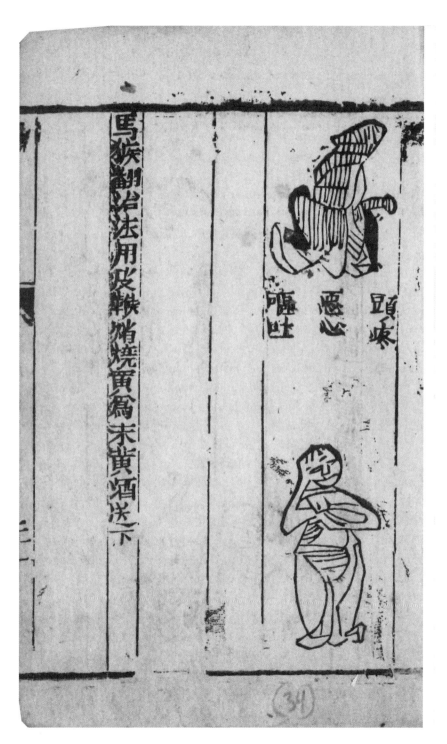

馬疾翻治法用沒鞦帶燒黃為末黃酒送下

頭疼
惡心
嘔吐

P35. Turtledove Therapy
Banjiu fan zhifang 斑鳩翻治方

Presenting Symptoms: Whining. Cold Limbs. Body Shivering.
Qi zheng: Shenming, sizhi ju liang, hunshen zhanzhan.
其症：伸鳴，四肢俱涼，渾身戰戰。

Turtledove Therapy. Take one or two twigs from a turtledove nest and burn to ashes. Drink with yellow rice wine.
Banjiu fan zhifang. Yong banjiuwo yi er gen, shaohui. Huangjiu song xia.
斑鳩翻治方。用斑鳩窩一二根，燒灰。黃酒送下。

In researching turtledoves, I found that there is no taxonomic difference between a turtledove and a pigeon. They look very similar. Apparently the word dove came into the English language from Nordic languages, while pigeon came into English from the French. Their meat and bones are low in sodium and are good sources of protein, vitamin B6, iron, and zinc.

Are the presenting symptoms asthma? Are they severe cold or flu? Classical Chinese medicine often prescribes acupuncture to bring relief to asthma sufferers, but in this case the recommendation is to burn one or two twigs from a turtledove nest and have the patient drink the decoction.

The major nutrient components of edible bird nest are said to be carbohydrates and glycoproteins. One also finds essential trace elements such as calcium, sodium, magnesium, zinc, manganese, and iron. Most prominent of the nutritutional elements contained are carbohydrates, amino acids, and mineral salts. The topic is studied in: Nurfatin Mohd Halimi, Zalifah Mohd Kasim, and Abdul Salam Babji, "Nutritional Composition and Solubility of Edible Bird Nest (Aerodramus fuchiphagus)," *AIP* (American Institute of Physics) *Conference Proceedings,* 1614.476 (February 2014), DOI: 10.1063/1.4895243.

Bird nest is considered good for helping to relieve respiratory ailments such as asthma or chronic coughs because of its ability to clear away phlegm (*pitan* 辟痰). It contains proteins, amino acids, and minerals essential for healthy development.

其症伸腰

四肢俱痛

渾身戰慄

班鳩翻洽方用班鳩窩二根燒灰黄酒送下

P36. Severing Knife [Razor] Therapy
Liedao fan zhifang 列刀翻治方

Presenting Symptom: Both Hands on the Mouth.

Qi xing: Liang shou zai kou laomo.

其形：兩手在口撈摸。

Severing Knife [Razor] Therapy. Take the beak of a crane and burn it until it becomes very fine. Add it to yellow rice wine and drink it down.

Liedao fan zhifang. Yong laoguanbi, bi shao wei ximo. He huangjiu, yin zhi.

列刀翻治方。用老鶴鼻，鼻燒為細末。和黃酒，飲之。

To the degree this therapy is sympathetic medicine, the beak represents the ability of the crane to cut away and clear with its long and sharp beak. From that perspective, the decoction symbolizes the ability of the patient to cut away the mental blockages that are causing the patient to act as if frightened and uncertain of their surroundings. This logic would account for the therapy being labeled as severing knife therapy (*liedao fan* 列刀翻). Seeing a person putting their hands on each side of their head or on the cheeks could easily be interpreted as a mental condition, perhaps fear, certainly an emotion of distress. In classical Chinese medicine the emotions are linked to internal organs: anger with the liver (*ganzang* 肝臟), fear with the kidney (*shen* 腎), sadness and grief with the lung (*fei* 肺), and worry with the spleen (*pi* 脾).

Bird beaks are comprised of keratin. Recent research has resulted in using keratin leading to the development of a keratin-based biomaterials platform with applications in wound healing, drug delivery, and trauma. See Jillian G. Rouse and Mark E. Van Dyke, "A Review of Keratin-Based Biomaterials for Biomedical Applications," *Materials (Basel)* 3.2 (February 2010): 999–1014, DOI: 10.3390/ma3020999, PMCID: PMC5513517. Keratin is also discussed in P23.

The ground remains of a bird beak seems to have been suggested both for its chemical properties and for its symbolic implications. Bird beaks often contain free calcium phosphate, hydroxyapatite, and keratin-bound phospholipids. Calcium helps in the regenerating phases of healing. As a part of the bird that could pull away and tear open, it was possibly that symbolic action that brought beaks to the attention of medical practitioners in China. In that case it was symbolic of tearing out the affliction.

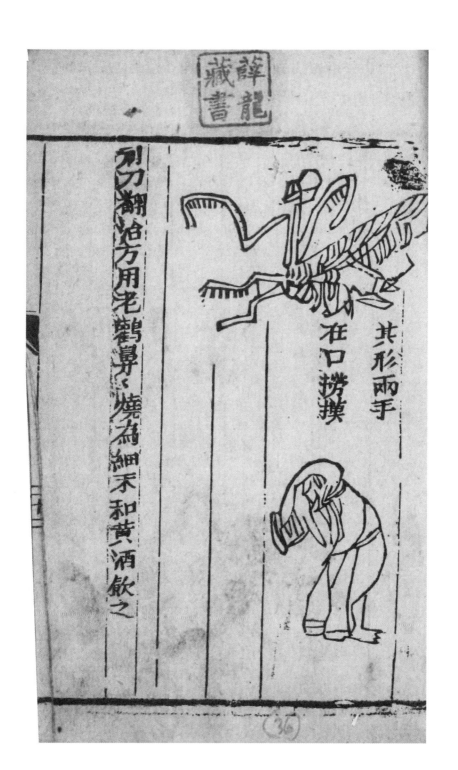

剡刀翻治方用老鸜鵒鼻、燒為細末、和黃酒飲之

其形兩手

在口撈摸

P37. Expelling the Topmost Pearl Therapy
Zhudingzhu fan 逐頂珠翻

Headache. Face Becomes Red.

Naozi tengtong. Lian fa hongse.

腦子疼痛。臉發紅色。

Expelling the Topmost Pearl Therapy. If prolonged [this condition] will be difficult to cure. Take the beak from a stork sitting in a grove of trees, burn the beak to ash. Add to rice wine and drink down. Relief will be achieved.

Zhudingzhu fan. Ri jiu nan zhi. Yong shu shu shang laoguanbi, bi duanhuang wei mo. Huangjiu song xia, ji yu.

逐頂珠翻。日久難治。用束樹上老鸛鼻，鼻煅黃為末。黃酒送下，
即愈。

The topmost pearl (*dingzhu* 頂珠; sometimes referred as the topmost pearl on Buddha, *fudingzhu* 佛頂珠), was a bead or button on the cap of a Qing Dynasty official to indicate his rank. The name of this therapy seems to indicate that some sort of pressure or weight is affecting the patient and needs to be removed. Having the patient drink the decoction of the ashes of a stork's beak with rice wine is prescribed. Pharmacist's shops in the market towns of 1860s China should have been stocked with cabinets of many drawers, each filled with a powder that was likely to be one of the items prescribed as a cure. Many Chinatowns in the United States have Asian pharmacies still stocked in this manner.

This prescription indicates that if the condition of the presenting symptoms of a headache and red face has been persistent for a long while, the causes of the affliction might be serious and the condition a difficult one to cure promptly. It is a recognition by the doctor that the effectiveness of this therapy might not be sufficient to effect a cure, possibly because accurately determining the cause of this condition in the patient is too difficult. See P55 for a listing of the use of bird beaks in this manual.

The illustration may be that of a female. Females are less frequently portrayed in early Chinese medical literature. No symbolic animal or insect was assigned to this therapy.

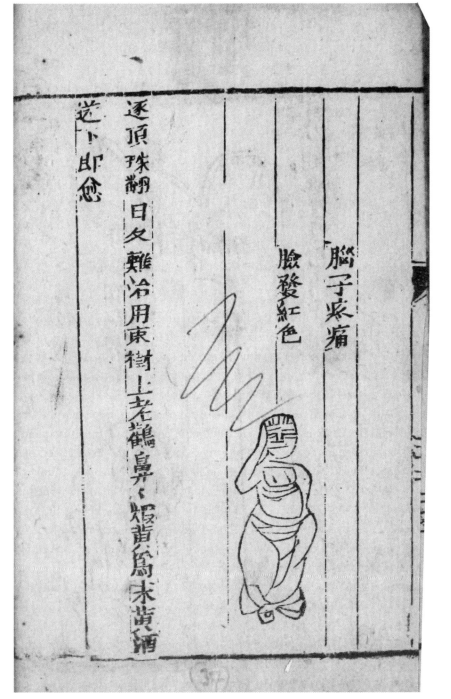

脑子疼痛

脸發紅色

逐顶珠翻日久難冷用東樹上老鸛鼻火煅青爲末黃酒

送下即愈

P38. Lack of Speech Therapy
Wuyu fan zhifang 無語翻治方

Presenting Symptom: Acquired Illness that Prevents Speaking.

Qi zheng: Debing bu yu.

其症：得病不語。

Lack of Speech Therapy. First insert a needle at the center of the forehead. Second [insert] a needle into the arch [underside] of the two feet. Third [insert] needles at the two Pools at the Bend.

Wuyu fan zhifang. Xian zhen tianmen yi zhen. Ci zhen liang jiaoxin. Youci zhen liang quchixue.

無語翻治方。先針天門一針。次針兩腳心。又次針兩曲池穴。

The presenting symptoms indicate a potentially serious illness that has taken over the patient. In confronting this problem, the Chinese doctor could resort either to an herbal decoction or acupuncture. In this case acupuncture is prescribed, and the points suggested for needles deal with the throat. First, a long-recognized pressure point on the forehead (*tianmen* 天門), above the area between the two eyebrows. This pressure point is called Hall of Impressions (*yintang* 印堂; sometimes in English the "third eye"), and often is used to treat anxiety, insomnia, frontal headache, and nasal obstruction. It is considered a non-channel accupuncture point, meaning that it does not lie on a meridian. It is sometimes listed as acupuncture point EM-2 or M-HN-3, depending on the classification scheme used. Second, along the kidney channel of the foot (*jiaoxin* 腳心) acupuncture point KI-08 in the ankle. It is on the meridian that helps to regulate blood flow. Third, the Pool at the Bend (*quchixue* 曲池穴) is at the crease that occurs when the elbow is bent. Acupuncture point LI-11 which is along the large intestine meridian. Several therapies in this manual recommend inserting acupuncture needles at the Pool at the Bend as an effective way to clear internal blockages. Also see P2.

    Blockages in the throat could be caused by wind (*feng* 風). Winds can be cold (*han* 寒) or hot (*re* 熱), moist (*ru* 濡) or dry (*zao* 燥). They can affect the lungs, liver, kidneys, intestines, stomach, or spleen. Whichever organ has been injured by a wind, the acupunture suggested here is designed to clear the blockages that have occurred in the flow of vital energy throughout the body, and the therapy focuses on the throat. This acupuncture point is also suggested in P2. A discussion of wind injuries to be cured by acupuncture and herbs are discussed in Mehrab Dashtdar et al., "The Concept of Wind in Traditional Chinese Medicine," *Journal of Pharmacopuncture* 19.4 (December 2916): 293–302, DOI: 10.3831/KPI.2016.19.030, PMCID: PMC5234349, PMID: 28097039.

No symbolic insect or animal was assigned to this condition.

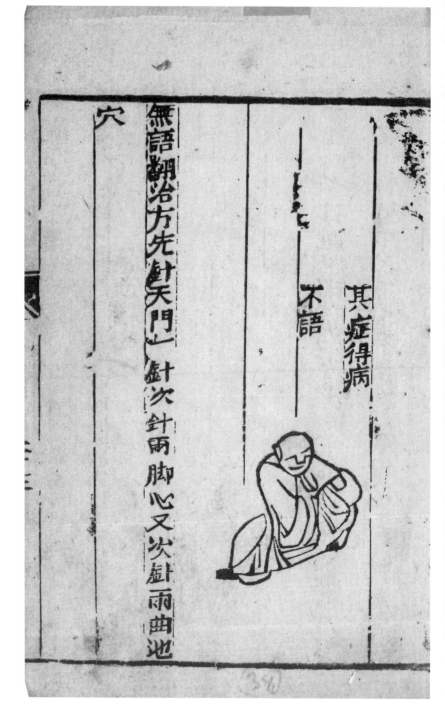

其症得病

不語

無語翻治方先針天門又針次針兩腳心又次針兩曲池

穴

P39. Blood on the Heart
Xue yongxin 血擁心

Blood on the heart for seven days, or pain. Needle the root of the tongue, jab it back and forth from front to back, for some relief. Another method is to steam a turnip to ashes, [followed by drinking] rice wine. Then use the needle to break the blisters under the tongue. Daub lightly with realgar water. Break open the red and black blisters, that will bring relief.

Xue yongxin qi ri, yong tuo huo tong. Zhen shegen shen xia, qianhou da, ji yu. You fang, yong zheng fu mo, huangjiu xia. You she xia you heipao, zhenpo. Xionghuang dian zhi, qianhou xin qing liao. Da chu hongheiquan, ji yu.

血擁心七日，擁脱或痛。針舌根身下，前後打，即愈。又方，用蒸菔末，黃酒下。又舌下有黑泡，針破。雄黃點之，前後心輕了。打出紅黑圈，即愈。

In classical Chinese medicine, the tongue (*she* 舌) is the sense organ related to the heart, and the condition of the heart can be seen by observing the tongue. When the heart is in balance, the tongue will be a healthy red color. If there is insufficient blood in the heart, the tongue may appear pale. If there is blood stagnation, the tongue will reflect this with a dark purple color or, in this case, with the appearance of "red and black blisters" (*hongheiquan* 紅黑圈).

The turnip is used for its ability to regulate *qi* 氣 and blood circulation. It helps to clear heat (*qingre* 清熱), resolve phlegm (*jietan* 解痰), and resolve dampness (*jieshi* 解濕). It is a *yang* 陽 tonic and detoxifies internal organs (*jiedu zangfu* 解毒臟腑) suffering from too much *yin* 陰. It is considered to be neutral in temperature, neither hot nor cold. The flavor is sweet, bitter, and pungent. Praise for turnips is in: Ahsan Javed et al., "Turnip (Brassica Rapus): A Natural Health Tonic," *Brazilian Journal of Food Technology* 22.5 (January 2019), DOI: 10.1590/1981-6723.25318.

This is another affliction not linked with an insect or symbolic animal.

血擁心

血擁心七日擁脫或痛針舌根身下並前后打即愈又方用
菜菔末黃酒下又舌下有黑泡針破雄黃塗之前后心輕
菜服出紅黑即愈

P40. Head Shaking, Navel is Also Extended
Touyao, duqi bian you pao fayu 頭搖，肚臍邊有泡發獄

This Affliction: Head Shaking. Navel is Also Extended.

Qi zheng: Touyao, duqi bian you pao fayu.

其症：頭搖，肚臍邊有泡發獄。

For bloated skin, the treatment [cure] can be done in one day. Use an acupuncture needle to break open the bloated blisters. To treat, take some ashes of realgar and smear them on. If [the affected area] gets bigger, it will be hard to cure.

Nuo pi ding, yi ri ji zhi. Yong zhen cipo yi nuo ding, shaohuang wei mo, dian zhi. Jiu ze yue zhang yue da, nan zhi.

挪皮疗，一日即治。用針刺破以挪疗，燒黃為末，點之。久則越長越大，難治。

In the presenting symptoms, the swelling of the navel brings on the nervous condition of shaking the head. This can be called a type of essential tremor. An essential tremor is a nervous system (neurological) disorder that causes involuntary and rhythmic shaking. The exact cause of the essential tremor is unknown. If there exist other more underlying causes, the tremor would not be labeled an essential tremor. The practitioner is aware that there might exist more serious or long term causes, thus the warning that "If [the affected area] gets bigger, it will be hard to cure."

The practitioners using this manual of quick remedies were always hopeful, I think, of quickly relieving the patient of their most troublesome presenting symptoms. Quick relief would boost the reputation of the practitioner, bringing in more business, and would greatly please the patient. Thus the important phrase at the beginning of this therapy: "For bloated skin, the treatment [cure] can be done in one day."

No symbolic insect or animal was assigned to this affliction. Does the artist's illustration suggest the patient may have reduced mental capabilities and appear to be vacantly smiling?

其症頭搖

肚臍邊有

泡發獄

挪皮疔一日即治用針剌破以榔疔燒黃爲末点之久則

越長越大難治

P41. The Blood Smells
Xuexing fuxin 血腥扶心

Presenting Symptom: A Lingering Rank Smell from Eating and Drinking.

Qi zheng: Yinshi shi ji wen xingqi.

其症：飲食時即聞腥氣。

The blood smells. There are purple blisters under the tongue. Puncture the blisters to cause bleeding, and apply a little realgar. If this does not relieve the condition, look carefully into the eye socket. If there are purple blisters there, use a pin to prick them, that will bring a cure.

Xuexing fuxin. She xia you ziding, cipo chuxue, xionghuang dian zhi. Ru bu yu, xikan shao yanwo nei, you zipao, zhenpo, ji yu.

血腥扶心。舌下有紫疔，刺破出血，雄黃點之。如不愈，細看少眼窩內，有紫泡，針破，即愈。

As with many of the afflictions presented by patients, in this case also it is recommended that a quick examination of the tongue should be made. Pistuals under the tongue filled with discolored blood indicate blockages of blood that must be relieved in order to allow the blood to flow smoothly. Classical Chinese medicine endorses the idea that acupuncture to the eyes can have a beneficial effect on sight by boosting overall visual acuity, reducing sensitivity to light, eliminating eye floaters, blurred vision, and dry eyes.

Using acupuncture on the eyes seems an especially delicate and potentially dangerous practice. Nevertheless, classical Chinese medicine did recommend acupuncture on the eyes if warranted, and there are claims for the results being better vision, brighter and healthy eyes. A common eye complaint is dry eyes, causing itchiness and irritation. The condition and acupuncture treatment is addressed in: Fabao Xu and Chenjin Jin, "Acupuncture and Ocular Penetration," *Ophthalmology* 128.2 (February 2021): 217, DOI: 10.1016/j.ophtha.2020.09.024.

But in this case one of the presenting symptoms is bad breath, which can be caused by problems with the digestive system. In modern medical analysis this could result from a bacterial infection in the intestine which, according to Chinese traditional medicine, would indicate an increase in pathogenic heat-related conditions. The eye is related to the liver (*ganzang* 肝臟). The liver regulates the body's blood sugar (*xuetang* 血糖). If toxins build up in the bloodstream, one result can be a foul-smelling breath. So if the problem is not simply one of interrupted blood flow, a problem with toxins in the intestines could be the cause and clearing the flow in the eyes could have a positive effect on the intestines.

No symbolic insect or animal was assigned to this affliction. Does the artist's illustration suggest this is just a case of human over-indulgence?

其症飲食

時即聞腥

氣

血腥扶心舌下有紫疔刺破出血雄黄點之如不愈細看

少服窩內有紫泡尉破即愈

P42. Elephant Therapy
Xiang fan zhifang 象翻治方

The Afflicted Has a Runny Nose Causing Distress and Occasional Dizziness.

Bingzhe liubi, xinteng, shimi.

病者流鼻，心疼，時迷。

Elephant Therapy. Puncture both shoulders and the belly with an acupuncture needle, use moxibustion to draw blood. Then apply a little realgar water after bleeding begins.

Xiang fan zhifang. Yong zhen tiao liang jian du, jiu chuxue. Xionghuang dian zhi.

象翻治方。用針挑兩肩肚，灸出血。雄黃點之。

A 1916 printed version of this medical recipe collection recommends needling "the shoulders and the rectum" (*tiao liang jian gang* 挑兩肩肛). Notice the similarity of the characters for belly and rectum. My copy of the text on which this translation is based, appears to have the word *du* 肚 for belly, rather than *gang* 肛 for rectum.

This medical problem was probably called the Elephant Therapy (*Xiang fan* 象翻) because elephants have a long nose or trunk as a prominent aspect of their anatomy. The human patient would be suffering extreme discomfort by having a constantly runny nose, as if the nose were enlarged into a long trunk? Runny nose (*liubi* 流鼻) is medically called rhinorrhea, meaning a continuous discharge of mucus from the nose, usually due to infection or allergy resulting in an excessive mucus secretion from the nose.

Among the techniques that can be used to quickly draw blood to the surface of the body and to thus promote a smooth flow of blood within the body, useful also for relieving stress and pains in the body, is moxibustion (*aijiu* 艾灸). This is the practice of stimulating acupuncture points by heating them through heating mugwort leaves (*aiye* 艾葉) and placing the burning leaves over the acupuncture point. Cupping (*baguan* 拔罐) is the practice in which a small glass jar is placed on the body, often on the patient's back. A vacuum is formed by allowing heat and smoke from the mugwort to enter the jar, which is then cupped (placed on the body) over the acupuncture point. The vacuum inside the jar causes the body's skin to be drawn into the jar. This sometimes breaks the skin and draws blood. When men in Asia remove their shirts in the summer, one can often see the round circles of bruises on their back caused by a moxibustion treatment. This is sometimes called a cupping therapy. Moxibustion and cupping can be used to draw blood (*jiu chuxue* 灸出血) and so open the constricted channels involved.

Dizziness, another of the presenting symptoms, can be caused by excessive gas in the abdomen. The runny nose, a continuous discharge of mucus from the nose, indicates the body has been invaded by external pathogenic factors (*xieqi* 邪氣), resulting in a battle between the pathogenic factors and the body's immunity, called the vital *qi* (*zhengqi* 正氣). Acupuncture points on the shoulder called the Shoulder Well (*jianjing* 肩經) acupuncture point GB-21 is said to sweep phlegm (*qingtan* 清痰) and open the orifices (*kaikong* 開孔). It quickens all of the network vessels.

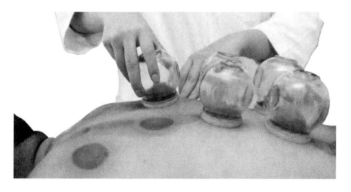

Cupping therapy (image by Kamonrat Meunklad)

象翔治方用鋮挑雨眉肚炎出血雄黃点之

病者流鼻

心疼時迷

P43. Lion Therapy
Shizi fan zhifang 獅子翻治方

Presenting Symptoms: Excitability, Headache, Large Blisters All over the Body.

Qi zheng: Xinhuang, toutong, hunshen qi dapao.

其症：心荒，頭痛，渾身起大泡。

Lion Therapy. Use an acupuncture needle to break the blisters, then daub with realgar water. Mix salt and vinegar with water and drink.

Shizi fan zhifang. Yong zhen cipo dapao. Xionghuang dian zhi. Yong yan cu shui, yin zhi.

獅子翻治方。用針刺破大泡。雄黃點之。用鹽醋水，飲之。

The word *pao* 泡 could be translated as swellings, distention, protrusions, or blisters. Blisters all over the body can be caused by many factors. Some are a fairly passing phenomenon, while others could be the sign of a more severe condition. Skin discomfort accompanied by a headache is not uncommon. In general, the culprit here seems to be heat (*re* 熱) and therefore the need to clear the heat (*qingre* 清熱), in this case through the use of acupuncture needles. Perhaps it is called the Lion Therapy because the lion is often depicted in China as having a mane of tight curls around his neck, imitating the sores of the patient's body?

Among Chinese symbolic ritual items are stone lion guardians (*shishi* 石獅) that are placed at the entrance of a building on either side of the gate, or at the base of a staircase. English speakers sometimes call them "*fu* dogs." Probably the word "*fu*" meant good fortune (*fu* 福) and their small size gives them a resemblance to dogs rather than to lions.

A propensity to continued excitability is not a normal human condition, so medical

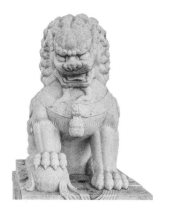

Fu dog
(adapted from image by "Mdy66," CC BY-SA 4.0)

tests have been carried out to see if acupuncture can have positive effects in reducing this condition. In this case the use of needles is only to break the blisters, but findings show that the symptoms can be relieved by the use of acupuncture. See Y. L. Lo and S. L. Cui, "Acupuncture and the Modulation of Cortical Excitability," *NeuroReport* 14.9 (July 1, 2003): 1229–1231.

其症心荒

頭痛渾身

起大泡

獅子翻治方用針刺破大泡雄黃点之用塩醋水敷之

P44. Cat Therapy
Mao fan zhifang 貓翻治方

Presenting Symptoms: The Nose and Two Hands Scratch and Embrace the Ground.

Qi xing: Bitun, liang shou naodi yongxin.

其形：鼻吞，兩手撓地擁心。

Cat Therapy. Pierce both temples with an acupuncture needle, drawing blood. Then drink realgar with yellow rice wine.

Mao fan zhifang. Zhen liang binjiao, chuxue. Zai yong xionghuang jiu, yin zhi.

貓翻治方。針兩鬢角，出血。再用雄黃酒，飲之。

The acupuncture points at the temples are called the Greater Yang (*taiyangxue* 太陽穴), EX-HN5. In accupuncture classifications this is known as an "extra point." It can be used to allieviate headache or toothache. Piercing the extra points with an acpuntcture needle and drawing blood should serve to disperse wind (*qufeng* 祛風) and dissipate heat (*huanre* 換熱), to clear the head (*qingnao* 清腦) and brighten the eyes (*mingyan* 明眼).

In this case the presenting symptoms have the patient acting like a cat moving close to the ground. Although this condition could have concerning internal causes, the immediate effect of acupuncture should be to have the afflicted person return to more normal behavior and posture. Some research on this accupuncture point is in Ya-Ting Lee, "Principle Study of Head Meridian Acupoint Massage to Stress Release via Grey Data Model Analysis," *Evidence-Based Complementary and Alternative Medicine* (2016), DOI: 10.1155/2016/4943204, accessed May 20, 2021.

其形鼻吞

兩手揣地

撚心

猫獬治方針兩髮角出血再用雄黃酒飲之

P45. Mouse Therapy
Laoshu fan zhifa 老鼠翻治法

There Are Mouse Shaped Abscesses on the Neck or Chest.

Bozi huo xiongqian qi ru laoshu chuangxing.

脖子或胸前起如老鼠瘡形。

Mouse Therapy. Stir-fry a cat's front paws to ashes, [along with] lime, mix with sesame oil and rub in.

Laoshu fan zhifa. Yong maoqianzhao, shihui, chao huang wei mo, xiangyou he cha.

老鼠翻治法。用貓前爪、石灰，炒黃為末，香油和搽。

The word *laoshu* 老鼠 can mean either a rat or a mouse in the label of this affliction. The method of stir-frying is to toss materials in a heated wok (*guo* 鍋) and stir them repeatedly while cooking. When preparing medicines in this manner, however, the cooking is dry frying and oil is not usually used. A concise description of this practice is in Nigel Wiseman and Andrew Ellis, *Fundamentals of Chinese Medicine* (Brookline, MA: Paradigm Publications, 1995), p. 491. This is a translation with annotations of *Zhongyixue jichu* 中醫學基礎 (*Fundamentals of Chinese Medicine*, 1985).

Using a cat's paws to remove an affliction that brings on a resemblance to a mouse seems to clearly be a case of sympathetic medicine. Perhaps the idea of saying the patient's face resembles that of a rat is because the patient might have a tendency to purse (pucker) the lips, making the mouth smaller and the nose seem more prominent? Similar to pouting (*juezui* 撅嘴)? This is not depicted in the artist's illustration.

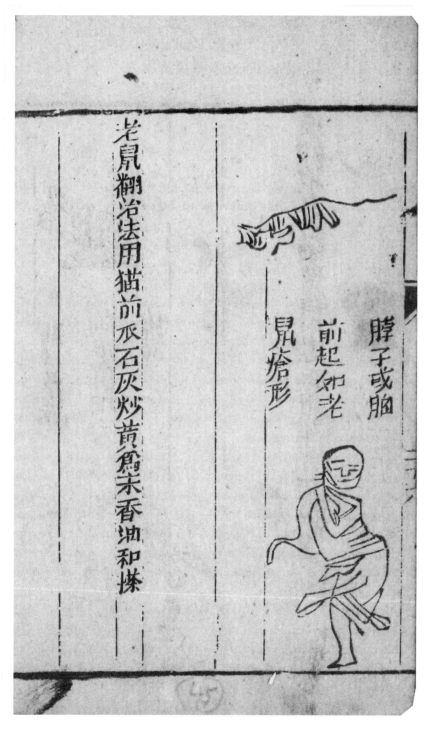

老鼠翻咬法用猫前爪石灰炒黄為末香油和搽

脖子或胞

前起如老

鼠瘡形

P46. Eagle Therapy
Ying fan zhifa 鷹翻治法

Snapping the Lips, Heartburn, Dizziness.

Juezui, xinteng, hunmi.

撅嘴，心疼，昏迷。

Eagle Therapy. Prick the arm and the leg [where they bend] with a needle. Bend [back and forth] until blood appears. Daub with realgar.

Ying fan zhifa. Yong zhen ci bowan, tuiwan, chuxue. Yi xionghuang dian zhi.

鷹翻治法。用針刺胳彎、腿彎，出血。以雄黃點之。

The word snapping the lips (*juezui* 撅嘴) listed as among the presenting symptoms can be taken as the expression of a person who is distressed or uncomfortable. Heartburn (*xinteng* 心疼) can result from stomach acid that causes a burning pain in the chest or throat, and leaves a sour taste in the mouth. Chinese doctors considered heartburn as a manifestation of disharmonies in the functions of the stomach (*wei* 胃) and liver (*ganzang* 肝臟). The goal of the basic treatment is to restore a balance between the liver and stomach to optimize their normal functioning.

Medical practitioners, in China when this manual was being circulated and equally at present, realize there is a connection between illness and disease and emotional health. Emotional health has always been seen as an integral part of Chinese medicine since the internal organs have a connection with the emotional, mental, and spiritual functioning of the body. Emotions are often expressed through facial expressions, in this case that snapping the lips. Emotions that are intense, prolonged, or repressed can inhibit the flow of *qi* 氣 to the internal organs.

As regards naming this the Eagle Therapy, keep in mind that the eagle eats its prey by pricking at it with its beak and then bending its head back to pull out the prey's insides, similar to the pricking of the shoulders and leg and then bending them back and forth to draw blood from the places where the needles were inserted.

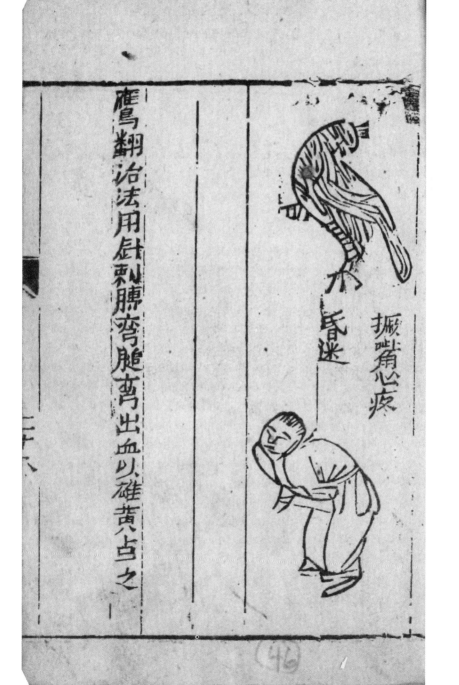

鷹鳥翻治法用針刺膘齊腿弯出血以雄黄占之

振嘴心疼

不昏迷

二十八

P47. Duck Therapy
Yazi fan zhifa 鴨子翻治法

Stiff Jaw, Shaking of the Head.

Banzui, yaotou.

板嘴，搖頭。

Duck Therapy. Pierce throat with a needle and after some bleeding the condition will be cured.

Yazi fan zhifa. Yong zhen, yanhou chuxue, ji yu.

鴨子翻治法。用針，咽喉出血，即愈。

There is no question that a clenched jaw will cause the facial muscles to ache and even the neck to feel strained. Tightness of the jaw can result from stress, anxiety, or injury. Too much chewing can also bring on this result. Involuntarily shaking the head could also be brought on by stress or anxiety. The condition might have been described as similar to the walking of a duck which frequently bobs its head on its long neck as it walks.

This therapy suggests a quick way to clear the blocked flow of blood and the tense muscles by a simple method. Acupuncture can also be recommended. In one clinical atricle this condition was described: "Myofascial pain is characterized by localized, hypersensitive spots in palpable taut bands of muscle fibers (myofascial trigger points). These trigger points may be due to muscle overload from trauma or repetitive activities that cause abnormal stress on specific muscle groups. Clinically, patients complain of tenderness, headaches, restricted movement, and muscle stiffness and weakness." See Yoshi F. Shen et al., "Randomized Clinical Trial of Acupuncture for Myofascial Pain of the Jaw Muscles," *Journal of Orofacial Pain* 23.4 (Fall 2009): 353–359, PMCID: PMC2894813, NIHMSID: NIHMS209743, PMID: 19888488.

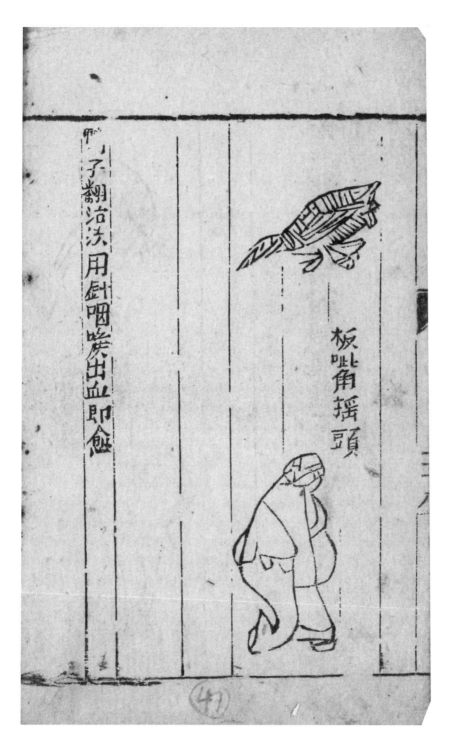

板咂角搖頭

蛉子翻治法用針咽喉出血即愈

P48. Chicken Therapy
Jizi fan 雞子翻

Presenting Symptom: Like a Sick Chicken, Unable to Remain Calm.

Xing ru bing ji, xinhuang buning.

形如病雞，心荒不寧。

Chicken Therapy. Take the membrane of a chicken gizzard and roast to ashes. Drink down with wine.

Jizi fan. Yong jineijin, lu huang wei mo. Jiu song xia.

雞子翻。用雞內金，爐黃為末。酒送下。

The basics of classical Chinese medicine are to maintain a balance in life forces and ensure the smooth flow of vital energy throughout the body. The presenting symptoms in this case are like an affliction of modern society: anxiety disorder. The afflicted person cannot remain calm and contented. By defining the patient's condition as like that of a constantly moving and jerking chicken, an antidote with sympathetic properties might be a chicken gizzard in this case ingested with rice wine.

Chicken gizzards (*jineijin* 雞內金) are a common Chinese medicine. It is actually the membrane of a chicken gizzard. Once injested it travels through the spleen (*pi* 脾), stomach (*wei* 胃), small intestine (*xiaochang* 小腸), and bladder (*pangguang* 膀胱) meridians. It has a yellow color with a sweet taste and has a tonic effect by being credited with slowing down acute reactions and to detoxify (*jiedu* 解毒) the body. The chicken gizzard will be able to replenish qi (*tianqi* 添氣) and blood (*tianxue* 添血). Some claim this will aid in reproductive problems. Modern research suggests that humans secrete more gastric juices and have better digestion after eating chicken gizzard. The basic problem of the patient may have been as simple as a case of food stagnation (*shizhi* 食滯).

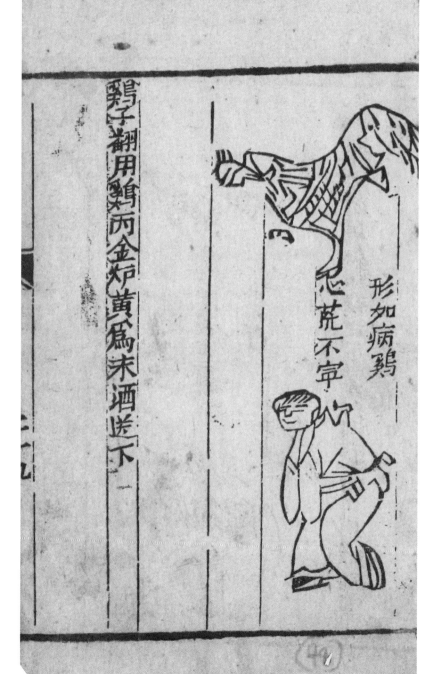

形如病雞

忘荒不宁

雞子翻用雞丙金炉黃為末酒送下一

P49. Magpie Therapy
Xique fan zhifa 喜雀翻治法

Distress and headache, with pains all over the body. Purple blisters under the tongue.

Xinteng touteng, yanhei, hunshen teng. She xia you ziding.

心疼頭疼，眼黑，渾身疼。舌下有紫疔。

Magpie Therapy. Use a needle to prick the purple blisters under the tongue. Sprinkle on that some realgar water. Then drink realgar wine for relief.

Xique fan zhifa. Yong zhen cipo shexia ziding. Xionghuang dian zhi. Zai yin xionghuang jiu, ji yu.

喜雀翻治法。用針刺破舌下紫疔，雄黃點之。再飲雄黃酒，即愈。

This therapy is translated as Magpie Therapy, but in the manual it is written with the word for "sparrow" (*que* 雀), with the expression "happy sparrow" (*xique* 喜雀). In Chinese a sparrow is usually referred to as *maque* 麻雀, which is not considered as a symbol of good luck and fortune. My advisor Dr. Stone Chen 陳實 has suggested I translate this as "magpie" (*que* 鵲). Both words are pronounced the same in standard Chinese. The figure in the illustration is smiling and appears happy (*xi* 喜).

The magpie is a small bird, often chirping and flitting about. In China it was a popular bird among elder men who kept them in hand-held cages in order to enjoy their singing. The cages might be carried to a park where other elders also had their magpies nearby, and the men would chat while the birds filled the air with song. This custom can still be seen in Chinese city parks. Some magpies have black and white feathers, while many magpies in Asia have predominantly blue or green colored feathers. The magpie is considered a symbol of good luck and good fortune. It is said that magpies can recognize human faces and distinguish the humans who are kind to them.

In this case of weakness and general distress in the patient, the Magpie Therapy is prescribed. The simple act of piercing the constricted blood in the blisters (*ding* 疔) under the tongue of the human patient, dabbing on a little realgar, then drinking some realgar is prescribed. The goal is to remove the pathogens (*xie* 邪) harming the body's channels, but to not go beyond that point because continuing this therapy could harm the right *qi* (*zhengqi*正氣) needed to keep the system strong since realgar is acidic and a source of highly toxic inorganic arsenic. Treatment should cease as soon as the purpose is achieved.

It is assumed the realgar will enter the kidney (*shen* 腎), lung (*fei* 肺), and bladder (*pangguang* 膀胱) meridians where it can strengthen *yang* 陽 and replenish essence (*jing* 精). There is a type of acupuncture called sparrow pecking (*quezhuo jiu* 雀啄灸), in which the acupuncture needle briefly pokes the skin and is then pulled out, similar to a sparrow pecking at corn. The purpose of the treatment is to is increase blood flow through muscles. See Hisashi Shimbara et al., "Effects of Manual Acupuncture with Sparrow Pecking on Muscle Blood Flow of Normal and Denervated Hindlimb in Rats," *Acupuncture in Medicine* 26.3 (October 2008): 149–159, DOI: 10.1136/aim.26.3.149.

心疼頭疼

紫疔

疼舌下有

眼黑渾身

即愈

壽字雀翻治法用剗剌破舌下紫疔雄黃點之再敕雄黃酒

P50. Bee Therapy
Fengmi fan zhifafang 蜜蜂翻治方

Sounds from the Throat. Nausea. Vomiting and Diarrhea. Purple Blisters under the Tongue.

Kengsheng buduan. Exin. Shangtu xiaxie. She xia you ziding.

吭聲不斷。惡心。上吐下瀉。舌下有紫疔。

Bee Therapy. Use a needle to pierce the purple blisters, then daub on salt.

Fengmi fan zhifang. Yong zhen cipo ziding, yi xiao yan dian zhi.

蜜蜂翻治方。用針刺破紫疔，以小鹽點之。

It seems a universal human reaction that when vomiting takes place, everyone knows that something is wrong. The Chinese have been studying vomiting and its causes for centuries. In this case the distress under the tongue is an indication of the internal forces causing the stomach to erupt, i.e. interrupted blood flows create purple blisters under the tongue.

Here is the way vomiting is described in terms of Chinese traditional medicine: "Vomiting is a common clinical symptom in which the conditions associated with impaired homeostasis and *qi* 氣 flow ascend reversely, acid upflow (*fansuan* 泛酸) within the stomach, resulting in the expulsion of the stomach's contents through the mouth. The stomach . . . is primarily responsible for receiving and digesting food and liquid, and its *qi* typically flows downward. Various unfavorable conditions associated with the environment, food, mental health, or physiological stress can compromise the stomach, thereby leading to a loss of gastric homeostasis, which often triggers vomiting. However, regardless of external factors or internal weaknesses, the direct cause of vomiting is the loss of gastric homeostasis and the ascending *qi* flow." See Yang Ling, Dan Yang, and Wenlong Shao, "Understanding Vomiting from the Perspective of Traditional Chinese Medicine," *Annals of Palliative Medicine* 1.2 (July 2012): 143–160, DOI: 10.3978/j.issn.2224-5820.2012.07.03, accessed May 21, 2021, http://apm.amegroups.com/article/view/1040/1267.

吭声不断恶

心上吐下泻

舌下有紫疔

蜜蜂螫治方用針刺破紫疔以小盐点之

P51. Four-Legged Snake Therapy
Sizushe zhifang 四足蛇治方

Pulsating Like the Heart. Boil Under the Tongue and the Corner of the Mouth is Sore.

Chuxin zhanzhan. She xia you ziding. Yi you koujiao qiangying zhe.

偹心戰戰。舌下有紫疔。亦有口角強硬者。

Four-Legged Snake Therapy. Take a needle and pierce [the swollen tongue], to cause bleeding. Smear on tobacco tar.

Sizushe zhifang. Yong zhen tiaopo chuxue. Yanyou dian zhi.

四足蛇治方。用針挑破出血。煙油點之。

Note that in Mandarin Chinese, the written words of tongue (*she* 舌) and snake (*she* 蛇) are both pronounced as *she* and have the same (second) tone.

Archaeologists have discovered skeletons of a snake-like animal that in pre-historic times had four small limbs or legs. Its body was long and flexible like that of a snake and the supposition is that the animal could burrow into the ground by digging with its legs. This animal has been termed *tetrapodophis.* Pharmacists in Chinese medicine shops often use chests with many drawers containing all sorts of bones, dried herbs, and powders . . . the perfect place where one might find the bones or a powder made from the skeleton of a four-legged snake.

This prescription calls for the tongue to be pierced to draw some blood, thereby allowing the constricted blood in the internal system to continue to flow. In this prescription, the Chinese practitioner must have realized that nicotine can have a calming effect on a person who is agitated as well as decreasing the degree of pain felt on the tongue, a sensitive human organ. A link between deadening pain and tobacco or nicotine has been known for decades and many people the world over have employed tobacco in cases of medical intervention. Nicotine results in the release of endorphins, which is the body's version of opioids. Nicotine causes an increase in adrenal function (epinephrine, norepinephrine), which results in increased arousal and a concommitant decrease in pain perception.

Among Western medical professionals tobacco has been demonized, so that research on tobacco use is at present almost always cast in terms of its potentially harmful consequences, with an attempt to dismiss the possibility of positive medical effects. The anti-smoking subtext guiding research can be detected in this otherwise sound article: Joseph W. Ditre et al., "Pain, Nicotine, and Smoking: Research Findings and Mechanistic Considerations," *Psychological Bulletin* 137.6 (November 2011): 1065–1093, DOI: 10.1037/a0025544, PMCID: PMC3202023, NIHMSID: NIHMS324174, PMID: 21967450. In contrast, information on the calming effect of tobacco tar has been published in a blog by Harvard Medical School. See Sharon Levy, "Nicotine: It May Have a Good Side," *Harvard Health Publishing* (March 2014), https://www.health.harvard.edu/newsletter_article/Nicotine_It_may_have_a_good_side#:~:text=For%20someone%20who's%20agitated%2C%20nicotine,manner%20as%, accessed August 10, 2020.

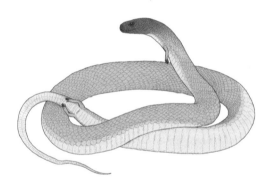

Tetrapodophis, the first known snake known to have four limbs
(image by SciFii, CC BY-SA 3.0)

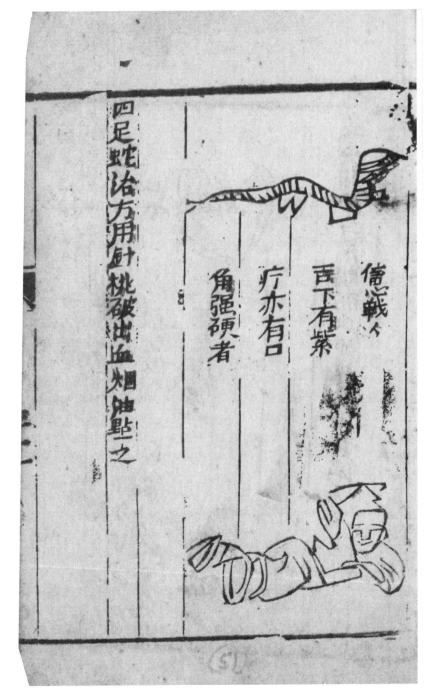

四足蛇治方用針桃破出血烟油點之

儵戰人

舌下有紫

疗亦有口

角强硬者

P52. Scorpion Therapy
Xiezi fan zhifang 蠍子翻治方

Presenting Symptoms: Crawling on the Ground. Legs Tapping the Ground Like a Scorpion Supported by a Curled Tail.

Qi xing: Padi, qiaodui, si xie juanwei, yongxin.

其形：爬地，敲腿，似蠍卷尾，擁心。

Scorpion Therapy. Take the claws from a house lizard or house gecko and burn to ashes. Mix with yellow rice wine and drink it down.

Xiezi fan zhifang. Yong xiehuzhao, lu huang wei mo. Huangjiu song xia.

蠍子翻治方。用蠍虎爪，爐黃為末。黃酒送下。

As in other presenting symptoms seen in this manual, the patient was acting in an unnatural way that resembled an animal or insect. The patient was exhibiting a type of spasm, possibly because of epilepsy, as they fell to the ground. In this case a portion of a common medicine called the claws of a house lizard (*xiehuzhao* 蠍虎爪) was prescribed as an antidote. Modern studies have analyzed the chemical elements of the house lizard, which include carnosine, choline, carnitine, guanine, protein, cholesterol, 14 amino acids, 18 kinds of trace elements, 5 types of phospholipid components, and 9 versions of fatty acids. These creatures have long been accepted as medicially beneficial by classical Chinese medicine.

Among the medical conditions that can be treated by the house lizard are epilepsy, seizures, and stroke. All of these can cause muscular spasms as exhibited by the patient in this desciption.

According to phamacologists in China, this medicine is used to address medical conditions where the body is expressing serious reactions to some cause. It can be used to treat apoplexy (*zuzhong* 卒中) and paralysis (*tanjifeng* 癱疾風), subdue endogenous (internal) wind (*neiyinfeng* 內因風), dispel toxins (*jiedusu* 解毒素), and settle convulsions (*dingjing* 定痙). These are the reactions being exhibited by the patient in the Scorpion Therapy scenario. Most pharmacies in China in the 1860s had dried house lizards for sale, just as they do in many areas of Asia today. They are often prescribed among remedies to relieve serious medical conditions.

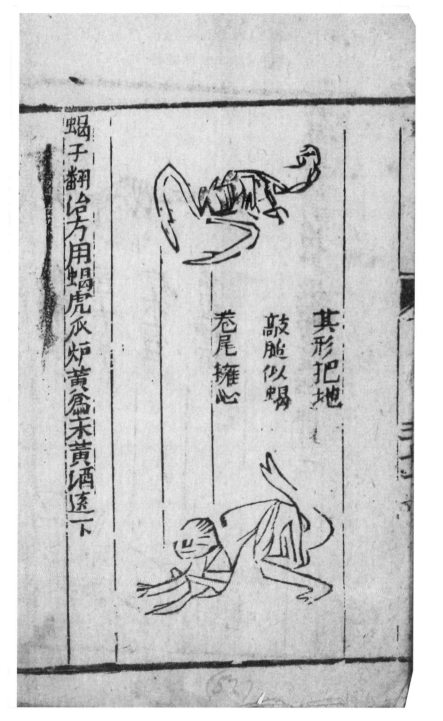

其形把地

敲腮似蝎

卷尾攅心

蝎子翻咬方用蝎虎瓦炉黄爲末黄酒送下

P53. House Lizard [Gecko] Therapy
Xiehu fan zhifang 蠍虎翻治方

Shaking the Head. Tremor in the Hands. Purple Blisters under the Tongue.

Yaotou baishou. She xia you ziding.

搖頭擺手。舌下有紫疔。

House Lizard [Gecko] Therapy. Using a needle to prick the blister. Daub on a little realgar.

Xiehufan zhifang. Yi zhen cipo ding. Xionghuang dian zhi.

蠍虎翻治方。以針刺破疔。雄黃點之。

This therapy is described as House Lizard or Gecko Therapy because the patient's symptoms made them sort of resemble a house lizard. But the prescribed therapy has nothing to do with a house lizard because it recommends acupuncture using needles. The symptoms of "shaking head, tremor in the hands, and purple blisters under the tongue" are related to a neurological disease, or maybe from high blood pressure or a tumor? In classical Chinese medicine this would be considered a blockage (*bi* 閉) in the body, meaning that the *qi* 氣 and the blood (*xue* 血) could not flow well. Or there imight be a heat toxin (*redu* 熱毒) in the body. That is probably why the therapy suggested acupuncture to release some blood and then realgar (*xionghuang* 雄黃) to detoxify (*jiedu* 解毒).

Geckos are small lizards found in warmer climates throughout the world. It is said that the English word gecko comes from the Indonesian-Malay word *gēkoq*, which imitates sounds made by some species. The name given to this set of presenting symptoms might have been derived from watching a gecko as it moved its head from side to side in search of food. The gecko has a long pointed tongue that it repeatedly seems to spit out and draw back quickly which may have been why this name was given to the acupuncture therapy of quickly pricking with the needle.

This therapy does not speculate on the cause of the patient's affliction. But an important report from 2008 suggests using the gecko in cancer treatment. The report reads in part, "Chemotherapy, one of the major methods to treat cancer in Western medicine at present, has a poor selectivity and strong toxic and side effects, thus influencing its anticancer effect. In the past 40 years, Chinese experts have gained remarkable achievements in cancer treatment by integrating TCM (Traditional Chinese Medicine) with chemotherapy. Now a research group in China has found that Gecko powder can inhibit EC9706 and EC1 growth and proliferation. The research team, led by Prof. Wang from Henan University of China, showed that Gecko could not only reinforce immunity of organisms but also induction of tumor cell apoptosis and the down-regulation of protein expression of VEGF and bFGF." See F. Liu et al., "Antitumor Effect and Mechanism of Gecko on Human Esophageal Carcinoma Cell Lines in Vitro and Xenografted Sarcoma 180 in Kunming Mice," *World Journal of Gastroenterology* 14.25 (2008): 3990–3996, http://www.wjgnet.com/1007-9327/14/3990.asp, DOI: 10.3748/wjg.14.3990.

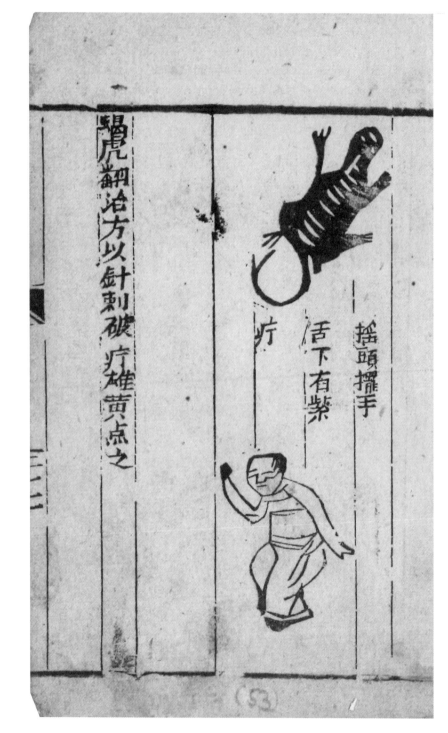

搖頭擺手

舌下有紫

疔

治方以針刺破疔雄黄点之

P54. Millipede Therapy
Youzi fan zhifang 蚰子翻治方

Falls to the Ground Holding the Chest. Distress. Hands on the Cheeks, Legs are Bent.

Fudi yongxin. Xinteng. Liang shou pengsai, qutui.

覆地擁心。心疼。兩手捧腮，屈腿。

Millipede Therapy. Use the herb *Geranium wilfordii Maxim*, and burn it to ashes. Drink it with yellow rice wine.

Youzi fan zhifang. Yong laoguanzui ke. Lu huang wei mo. Huangjiu xia.

蚰子翻治方。用老鸛嘴科。爐黃為末。黃酒下。

While the typical name for a centipede in Chinese is *wugong* 蜈蚣, the insect referred to in this therapy should be classified as a millipede (*you* 蚰). The millipede is a thin creature somewhat resembling a worm. The body is composed of many small body sections. Each section has a double pair of legs. It resembles a centipede, which has one pair of legs on each body section.

While the centipede is used for medicinal purposes and gave its name to the recipe P60 below, it appears the millipede is not used for this purpose. The millipede does not bite or sting, but gives off a toxic substance when attacked, causing in humans burning, blisters, intense itching, and the skin turning brown. Remarks on the millipede are in Petra Sierwald et al., "Current Status of the Myriapod Class Diplopoda (Millipedes): Taxonomic Diversity and Phylogeny," *Annual Review of Entomology* 52.1 (2007): 401–420, DOI: 10.1146/annurev.ento.52.111805.090210, PMID: 17163800.

The herb *laoguanzui* 老鸛嘴 recommended in this case is *Geranium wilfordii Maxim.* It is usually listed in the Chinese Pharmacopeia as the *Geranii Herba.* This edible herb is used to treat spasms and limb numbness, the conditions being exhibited by the patient in this case. Further uses include treating rheumatism, infectious diseases, dermatosis and tumors. It is also known as *Herba Erodii.* All of these names indicate the herb is extracted from the geranium family of plants. Among this species a common version in North America is called the Carolina Cranesbill, and the word "cranesbill" seems to be a translation of the Chinese name for this herb, *guanzui* 鸛嘴.

覆地掩心

心疼兩手

子捧脇屈腿

子翻治方用老鸛嘴科爐黃兔末黃酒下

P55. Cicada Therapy
Qiuchan fan zhifang 秋蟬翻治方

Muscles of the Limbs Turn Blue. Tendons at Back of Head Turn Purple.

Sizhi jin qing. Naomo shao hou you zijin.

四肢筋青。腦抹勺後有紫筋。

Cicada Therapy. Prick the purple tendons with a needle. Use the herb *Geranium wilfordii Maxim* and burn to ashes. Daub this on the affected areas.

Qiuchan fan zhifang. Yi zhen cipo zijin. Yong laoguanzui, lu huang wei mo, dian zhi.

秋蟬翻治方。以針刺破紫筋。用老鸛嘴,爐黃為末,點之。

The herb *Geranium wilfordii Maxim* (*laoguanzui* 老鸛嘴) recommended in this case is the same as that in P54. In this case a version of acupuncture is also used, at least to prick the skin and then daub on the ashes of the burnt plant.

This affliction is called the cicada disease (*qiuchan fan* 秋蟬翻) and a cicada has a relatively short life span, perhaps indicating that the patient's affliction will soon be cured? This would align with the Chinese symbolism of the cicada, that it was a symbol for immortality and a religious symbol for reincarnation, leaving one's "old" life or body behind and starting fresh or "anew." See the explanation in P18 for more comments on cicada molting, which more specifically refers to the molted exoskeleton of a cicada.

The recommended herb is from the geranium family of plants. In this case the patient seems to be reacting to a severe condition and the doctor wants to quickly relieve the symptoms. But it is also known that the geranium can be used to relieve less serious but still annoying conditions such as sunburn, insomnia, and varicose veins. It can help to heal bruises, cuts and scrapes, and eczema. It is sometimes prescribed to treat hemorrhoids and nail fungus. It has long been considered a natural insect repellent including for ticks on humans or their pets.

The medical properties of geranium plants have long been recognized by both Asian and Western doctors. The following therapy (P56) also recommends a powder or ointment daubed on the afflicted area.

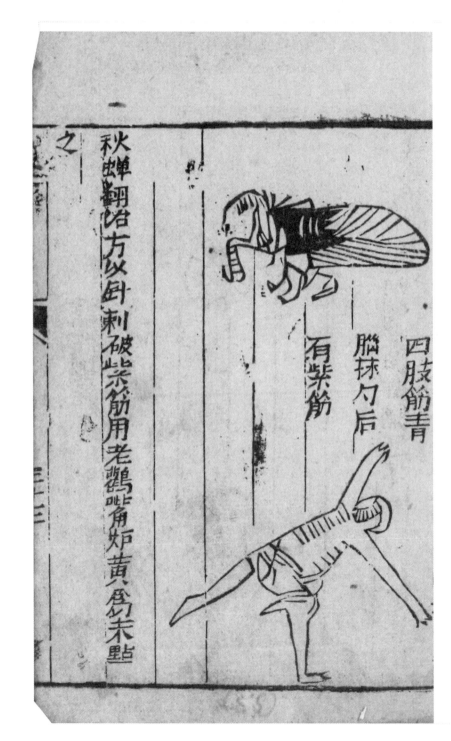

四肢筋青

腦抹勺后

有紫筋

秋蟬翅沿方以臥剌破紫筋用老鸛嘴角爐黃登幻未點

P56. Earthworm Therapy
Qiuyin fan zhifang 蚯蚓翻治方

Shaking Head and Buttocks. Vomiting and Diarrhea.

Yaotou baiwei. Shangtu xiaxie.

搖頭擺尾。上吐下瀉。

Earthworm Therapy. Use earthworm droppings and mix with yellow rice wine. Drink it down.

Qiuyin fan zhifang. Yong qiuyin fen, he huangjiu song xia.

蚯蚓翻治方。用蚯蚓糞，和黃酒送下。

Shaking the head and twitching the buttocks could be a reaction of nerves, but the vomiting and diarrhea indicate possible internal organ issues as well. Earthworms have been used as medicine to treat seizures caused by high fevers, to ease the pain of arthritic joints, to lower blood pressure, and to relieve blood stasis caused by fevers. In Western medicine the relief agents applied are referred to as antispasmodic, anti-inflammatory, and antipyretic. These are the calming results the patient appears to need and the earthworm therapy seems to have been effective for all of these maladies.

Earthworm has been a specific recommendation for disorders classified as true heat (*zhenre* 真熱), sometimes translated as full heat, which means an excessive manifestation of *yang* 陽. A very brief overview of the medical use of earthworms, though not making reference to these analytical categories, is in Yu Shen, "Earthworms in Traditional Chinese Medicine," *Advances of the 4th International Oligochaeta Taxonomy Meeting, Zoology in the Middle East, Supplementum 2* (Heidelberg: Kasparek Verlag, 2010), pp. 171–173.

搖頭擺尾

上吐下瀉

蚯蚓翻治方用蚯蚓糞和黃酒送下

P57. Mantis Therapy
Tanglang fan zhifa 螳螂翻治法

Head Bent to One Side. Distress. In a Stupor.
Touxie bu zheng. Xinteng. Hunmi.

頭斜不正。心疼。昏迷。

Mantis Therapy. Look at the elbow to see if it is discolored or broken. Use a hooked beak and burn it to ashes. Apply.
Tanglang fan zhifa. Kan bowan you zijin, tiaopo. Yong laozhaobi shaohui, dian.

螳螂翻治法。看膊彎有紫筋，挑破。用老爪鼻燒灰，點。

The herb recommended here "hooked beak" (*laozhaobi* 老爪鼻) was written in my manual used for translation. But my advisor Dr. Stone Chen feels it might in fact be the same herb recommended in P54 and P55 above, which was *Geranium wilfordii Maxim* (*laoguanzui* 老鸛嘴). We have not resolved this issue.

In the crook of the arm is an acupuncture point called Pool at the Bend (*quchixue* 曲池穴; this acupuncture point is also mentioned in the therapy of P2). It is a key point on the internal meridian, and for extreme internal issues it can be bled to relieve problems caused by evil (toxic) heat (*xiere* 邪熱) in the internal system. In this case a problem revealed in the area of this point on the body, combined with the presenting symptoms, indicate a possibly serious internal problem. The mantis (*tanglang* 螳螂) is used to clear problems with the bladder (*pangguang* 膀胱), kidney (*shen* 腎), and liver (*ganzang* 肝臟). The prepared ointment is daubed onto the area.

The patient appeared to be in a stupor because of the pathogen that had invaded the body. The many ways the internal organs could be invaded by an evil pathogen (*exie* 惡邪) are enumerated in a relaxed comic-book style in Damo Mitchell and Spencer Hill, *The Yellow Monkey Emperor's Classic of Chinese Medicine* (London: Singing Dragon, 2016).

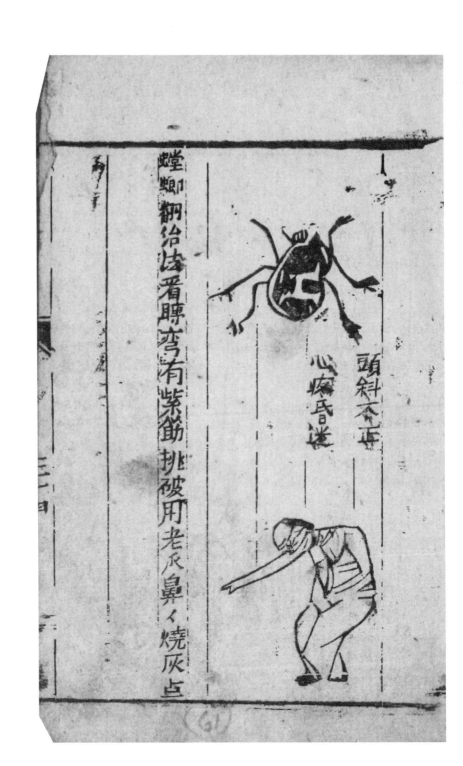

螳螂翻治法看脣弯有紫節挑破用老尿鼻人燒灰点

頭斜不正

心疼昏迷

三十四

P58. Mosquito Therapy
Wenzi fan zhifa 蚊子翻治法

The Mouth Spits Phlegm. In a Stupor.

Koutu niantan. Hunmi.

口吐黏痰。昏迷。

Mosquito Therapy. Use heated wine. [This to be used as an external medicine, applied to the pit of the stomach.] Strike the pit of the stomach with your hands until it becomes red, then stop.

Wenzi fan zhifa. Yong shaojiu pai xinkou, zhi hong zhushou.

蚊子翻治法。用燒酒拍心口，至紅住手。

As in the case of P57 above, the patient is acting strangely and as if not fully conscious, probably drooling at the mouth. The logic of analyzing the presenting symptoms must have been that the internal organs of the patient were desperately trying to cure the blockages of the vital forces in the body by causing a strange dizzy feeling and spewing out phlegm. Striking the lower belly until it looked like it had received numerous mosquito bites would jar loose the constrictions that were centered in the stomach as evidenced by the phlegm being expelled.

The stomach meridian (*weijing* 胃經) is placed at the intermediate abdominal wall, similar to the spleen meridian (*pijing* 脾經). From a cystic fibrosis perspective, they help track helical biodynamics because together they initiate the twisting movements which would cause the patient to move unsteadily as if in a stupor. The negative emotions linked to this meridian that need to be addressed are overwork, pensiveness, and worry.

口吐粘痰

昏迷

敗子翻治法用燒酒拍心口至紅佳乎

P59. Getting to the Heart [Cause] Therapy
Chuanxin fan fang 穿心翻方

Presenting Symptoms: Disturbed Personality. Mucus Discharge. Unable to Function in Society.

Qi xing: Xinshen buning. Touli. Tanyong. Buzhi renshi.

其形：心神不寧。頭立。痰湧。不知人事。

Getting to the Heart [Cause] Therapy. Using a pair of rotten [soft] wooden chopsticks, slap the eyebrows and abdomen.

Chuanxin fan fang. Yong xiumu zhuzi da meiquan ji pan quchi.

穿心翻方。用朽木箸子打眉全及盤曲池。

An important presenting symptom here is the mucus or phlegm (*tan* 痰) noticed by the doctor. Phlegm is always due to a pathology of fluids within the body. Many organs could be involved in this dysfunction, including the lungs (*fei* 肺), stomach (*wei* 胃), kidneys (*shen* 腎), and bladder (*pangguang* 膀胱). Emotional stress can lead to a *qi* deficiency (*qixu* 氣虛) or stagnation (*qizhi* 氣滯), sometimes both. Phlegm can obstruct the psychic spirit (*shen* 神). Obstruction of the *shen* causes a number of the other presenting symptoms observed in this case: mental confusion, strange behavior, and even manic behavior, all of these making the patient unable to function in society.

Striking with chopsticks is prescribed to shock this troubled system back into the normal flow of liquids and to restore balance, even if only temporarily. My comments above are based on a report by Giovanni Maciocia 馬萬里 in his article "Phlegm-Heat in Chinese Medicine," https://giovanni-maciocia.com/phlegm-hea/, accessed June 3, 2021. We find other examples in this manual where the simple act of striking the patient, with intent to "shock" and not to injure, is prescribed in P1, P4, and P8

No symbolic animal or insect was assigned to this therapy.

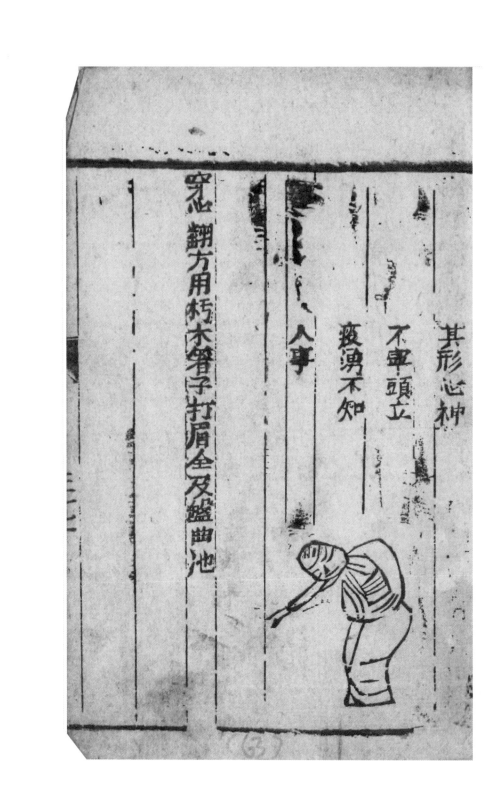

究翻方用朽木簪子打肩全及鑑曲池

其形心神

不卑頭立

疼湧不知

人事

P60. Centipede Therapy
Wugong fan zhifang 蜈蚣翻治方

Cold Sweat from the Head. Congestion. Spitting Yellow Phlegm. Purple Tendons on Both Sides of the Spine.

Tou chu lenghan. Yongxin. Tu huangshui. Jigu liang pang you zijin.

頭出冷汗。擁心。吐黃水。脊骨兩旁有紫筋。

Centipede Therapy. Use a needle to puncture the purple tendons. Daub on realgar.

Wugong fan zhifang. Yong zhen cipo zijin. Xionghuang dian zhi.

蜈蚣翻治方。用針刺破紫筋。雄黃點之。

Centipedes (*wugong* 蜈蚣) are often utilized in classical Chinese medicine. Centipedes are said to have an unpleasant odor and are somewhat salty in taste. They are usually boiled, dried in the sun, then ground into a powder for use in herbal preparations.

As a medicine centipedes are said to be reinvigorating. They are associated with the liver meridian (*ganjing* 肝經) and have pungent, warm, and slightly toxic properties. Its efficacies are to clear wind (*qingfeng* 清風) and spasms (*jingluan* 痙攣), and to dissipate toxins (*qusan dusu* 驅散毒素) and nodules (*jiejie* 結節), which are the presenting symptoms of the patient in this case. They can more specifically be used to counter the effects of epilepsy, stroke, cancer, tetanus, or rheumatoid arthritis. When used as medicine they are eaten dried, powdered, or after being steeped in alcohol.

In China, centipedes are sometimes skewered and deep fried or grilled and are sold at street vendor's stalls. I visited such a stall behind the Beijing Hotel (*Beijing fandian* 北京飯店) on Xiagongfu Street (*Xiagongfu jie* 霞公府街) in about 2007 when it was still an area of small family-owned businesses, like tailor shops and sundry goods. Both children and adults were surprised by the skewered centipedes on sale. Some of the insects were still struggling before being roasted. Many people turned away nervously, but others were buying the roasted centipedes because the stalls continued in business over the week I was in the city. Sometimes centipedes are submerged in liquor bottles because they add to the medicinal effect of the drink.

頭黑冷汗

擁心吐黃

水眷骨兩

旁有紫筋

蜈蚣翻治方用尉刺破紫筋雄黃點之

Extra Therapies

The following therapies P61 to P64 appear without illustrations in my copy of the manual and also in some other versions I have seen on the internet. In my manual, when they appear without illustrations, they are simply listed next to each other on the page. As they appear in translation below, they are labeled P61a, P61b, P61c, P61d, P61e, and P61f, which is the pattern followed through to and including the therapies on P62, P63, and P64.

Note that some of the recipes in this section use a pharmacist's mark 个 which is pronounced *qian*. The *qian* 錢 (dividing the *liang* used during the Republican period [1912–1949] by 10) was 3.7301 grams or 0.1316 ounce. The transliterations in this section write the character *qian* in place of the pharmacist's mark 个. Some versions of the available publications I have examined also transcribed the mark as the character for money (*qian* 錢).

Why was this collection of therapies often listed together at the end of the illustrated section of the publication and without illustrations? It could be that these afflictions can apply to women and children in many cases. Women and children were considered in a different category in the highly male-oriented thinking of the time. In contrast, the majority of therapies in this manual are illustrated by male figures and would seem to appear more often in adults.

P61a. Nine Types of Distress
Jiu zhong xinteng 九種心疼

Use the plant called Tree of Heaven and process it [fry it] into a powder. Each dose composed of three small portions. Drink this down with a ginger soup to effect relief.

Yong chouchunzi chao guo wei mo. Yi fu san qian. Jiangtang tiao xia, li xiao.

用臭椿子炒過為末。一服三个。薑湯調下，立效。

Three small portions (*san qian* 三个 [錢]) would equal about 11.19 grams or 0.40 ounce. The name "Tree of Heaven" (ailanthus altissima) in English sounds great, but the Chinese is closer to the truth, because with a direct translation the Tree of Heaven is called a Stinking Sumac (*chouchun* 臭椿). It releases a strong offensive smell particularly from its flowers. It is a rapidly growing deciduous tree native to China. It has an aggressive root system that can cause damage to pavement, sewers, and building foundations in urban areas.

Why was it ever called Tree of Heaven? It got this name perhaps because it is effective as a medicinal plant. The dried bark, stem, and root are used to act against a number of troublesome conditions. Among these are: diarrhea, asthma, cramps, epilepsy, fast heart rate, gonorrhea, malaria, and tapeworms. It has also been used as a bitter and a tonic. It alleviates damp heat (*shire* 濕熱). It is an astringent (*se* 澀) to stop leakage such as bleeding. It settles wind and stops coughs. The name of this therapy, Nine Types of Distress (*Jiu zhong xinteng* 九種心疼), could be translated as "All Types of Distress."

P61b. Empty the Secrets of the Heart
Daobao caoxin 倒飽饡心

Stir-fry medicated leaven into a powder. Each dose will be three small portions. Drink it down with yellow rice wine. That will bring relief.

Yong shenqu chao wei mo. Yifu san qian. Huangjiu song xia, li zhi.

用神曲炒為末。一服三个。黃酒送下，立止。

The character written as *cao* 饡 in the title is composed of the radical for food (*shi* 食) and the phonetic (*cao* 曹). This character is equivalent to the word "secret," or could refer to the tiny portions used as stuffing (*xian* 餡) in meat dumplings called *jiaozi* 餃子. This character *cao* 饡 is not found in many standard Chinese dictionaries these days. Three portions (*san qian* 三个) would equal about 11.19 grams or 0.40 ounce.

Medicated leaven is labeled *massa fermentata*. As the Latin name indicates, it is actually a mix of a variety of herbs, said to be a simple formula of wheat flour, bran, flowering pants, artemisia, and apricot. The mixture is covered by mulberry leaves and left to ferment. This sweet and pungent tasting herbal mix goes to the spleen (*pi* 脾) and stomach (*wei* 胃) meridians to strengthen the organs and improve digestion. It has been observed to help lower cholesterol and improve the appetite. This mixture should bring to the patient a general feeling of relief and well-being.

Apricot peel (*chenpi* 陳皮) was a frequently used ingredient in traditional medical recipes. Its presence in a decoction intended to calm and sooth a distressed patient is in Bao Xiangao 鮑相璈, *Raising the Dead and Returning Life: Emergency Medicine of the Qing Dynasty* (*Qisi huisheng* 起死回生), trans. Lorraine Wilcox (Portland, OR: Chinese Medical Database, 2012), pp. 160–161.

P61c. Regurgitation and Belching
Yege fanwei 噎嗝反胃

Make a dog go hungry for four days. Take millet feed and add it to the dog's droppings. Take clean and boiled rice gruel. Add to all this some aloe, and drink a portion slowly.

Ba gou gane si ri. Yong xiaomi wei zhi, deng la xia shi. Ba mi taojing zhu zhou, zai ru chenxiang mo yi qian chi.

把狗乾餓四日。用小米餵之,等拉下屎。把米淘淨煮粥,再入沉香末一个吃。

The aloe mentioned here is aloeswood (*chenxiang* 沉香), the powder of a dark resinous wood used in incense, perfume, and small carvings. This was probably intended to mask the taste of the mixture and to give it an overall pleasant flavor. After four days of only water, the doctor assumed the dog's stool would be fairly clear of food residue yet would contain the healing properties sometimes credited to animal dung. One portion (*yi qian* 一錢) equals 3.73 grams or 0.13 ounce.

Research on the medicinal properties of fecal matter has been published by Huan Du et al., "Fecal Medicines Used in Traditional Medical System of China: A Systematic Review of Their Names, Original Species, Traditional Uses, and Modern Investigations," *Chinese Medicine* 14.31 (September 2019), DOI: 10.1186/s13020-019-0253-x.

P61d. Vomiting Blood Because of an Internal Lesion Caused by Overexertion

Laoshang tuxue 勞傷吐血

Using the patient's own urine, add incense ash. Take two small doses for relief.

Yong ziji niao yi zhong, jia xiangmo er qian tiaofu, ji yu.

用自己尿一中，加香墨二个調服，即愈。

The best medicine for this condition will be a mixture that has a calming effect on the internal organs. The well-known Chinese pharmacopeia *Bencao gangmu* 本草綱目 recommends camphor (*zhangnao* 樟腦). It can expel wind (*feng* 風) and dampness (*shiqi* 濕氣), especially the evil wind (*fengxie* 風邪) in the heart and belly. It also kills parasites, promotes blood circulation, and alleviates pain. It can also mask the human urine taste, which may be the reason the fragrant ink (incense ash, *xiangmo* 香墨) is listed in this recipe. The phrase *erqian tiaofu* 二个調服 means to mix together two doses and drink it down. The two doses would be 7.46 grams or 0.26 ounce.

Camphor is used to make incense and to produce scents that seem to cleanse and protect. We probably know from general life that camphor is a warming agent, and it has an antiseptic effect on the skin. It has mildly local anesthetic properties. Its irritant effect is that it promotes blood circulation and increases mucosa secretion, which means it helps clear our sinus. A number of other herbs used to make incense have similar properties of being fragrant and calming.

P61e. Severe Toothache
Fenghuo yateng 風火牙疼

Use Sichuan pepper and mugwort. Regardless of the amount, fry them together. Place them in the mouth to stop [the pain].

Yong huajiao aihao. Buju duoshao, tong jian. Shukou, ji zhi.

用花椒艾蒿。不拘多少，同煎。束口，即止。

According to classical Chinese medicine, mugwort (*artemisia argyi, aihao* 艾蒿) leaf has bitter, pungent, and warm properties. It is associated with the liver (*gan* 肝), spleen (*pi* 脾), and kidney (*shen* 腎) meridians. It can warm the meridians and stop bleeding; it can dispel cold and stop pain. Mugwort is one of the herbs regularly used in moxibustion. Moxibustion (*jiu* 灸) is a method of heating specific acupuncture points on the body by burning an herbal material close to the skin. The mugwort is burned either in a cone-shaped pile, or on top of an acupuncture needle. In this prescription, the mugwort has been burnt to a powder and is placed in the mouth.

The Sichuan pepper (*huajiao* 花椒), sometimes called prickly ash, bark, or berry, are used in classical Chinese medicine. They have pungent and hot properties and are slightly toxic. When eaten it produces a tingling, numbing effect because of the presence of hydroxy-alpha-sanshool in the peppercorn. This plant is associated with the spleen (*pi* 脾), stomach (*wei* 胃), and kidney (*shen* 腎) meridians. Its main functions are to warm the spleen and stomach, and to stop pain. It is prescribed to treat vomiting, diarrhea, and stomach pain. In this case, by placing it in the mouth it should stop the toothache.

When I was a child and had a toothache, my parents let me suck on cloves (*dingxiang* 丁香) which has several properties similar to mugwort. My parents were unaware that cloves have been used in classical Chinese medicine since ancient times. Cloves are a warming or *yang*-energy herb that warms the stomach. Along with treating nausea and vomiting, the essential oil of the clove is used to reduce inflammation and kill pain, especially dental pain. As a child I disliked the taste of cloves, but now as an adult I rather like their pungent taste.

P61f. Intermittent Fevers/Malaria
Hanre nüezi 寒熱瘧子

Obtain a southeast-facing branch from a peach tree and boil it thoroughly [into a decoction]. Set that outside one night to let it get covered with dew. Drink it before the meal [on an empty stomach] and it will stop [the fevers].

Yong taoshu dongnan zhi, jian hao. Lu yi su, kongxin fu, li zhi.

用桃樹東南枝，煎好。露一宿，空心服，立止。

The presenting symptoms by the patient would be fevers and might not necessarily have been caused by malaria. Malaria fevers were widely known in China in pre-modern times, continuing into the twentieth century. The peach (*tao* 桃) tree has a strong symbolic meaning in Chinese culture. Its fruit is called the immortal peach (*xiantao* 仙桃) which is a symbol of longevity. Peach wood is known as immortal wood (*xianmu* 仙木) because it easily drives away evil spirits and troublesome ghosts.

Several parts of the peach tree can be used to prepare palliatives, including the tree bark, branches, the peach fruit, blossoms, kernels from the fruit, and the tree resin. For example, the kernels from a peach tree (*taoren* 桃仁) can treat blood stagnation (*xueyu* 血瘀) as a laxative for constipation from dryness and weakness. The peach fruit is considered a warm (*wen* 溫) herb that travels through stomach (*wei* 胃) and large intestine meridians (*dachangjing* 大腸經). It nourishes *yin* 陰 energy, activates blood circulation, and relieves night sweats.

A branch from a southeast-facing portion of the tree would be expected to be especially healthy since it would have received a maximum amount of possible sunlight. Fresh dew was considered a cleansing and strengthening agent in classical Chinese medicine. The Chinese have long considered the dew (*lu* 露) that forms on leaves and plants to be especially efficacious, providing both physical and emotional sustenance. Some ancient peoples took it as a mysterious substance appearing magically out of the night sky; it was first absent and then suddenly there, as if produced by nature's metamorphosis from dark to light. See Sara Crow, "Dew and Flower Essences," *Floracopia,* https://www.floracopeia.com/dew-and-flower-essences.

九種心疼　立効　用臭橘子、炒過爲末、一服三小、姜湯調下

倒飽饞心　用神曲炒爲末、一服三小、黄酒送下立止

噎隔反胃　米洗凈煑粥再入沈香末一小吃

　　把狗干屎四五丹、用小米裹之、等拉下屎把

勞傷吐血　用自己屎一中加香墨二小調服即於

風火牙疼　用花椒芝蔴不拘多少同並棗口即止

寒熱瘧子　用桃樹東南枝煎好露一宿空心服立止

P62a. Head Scabs on Children
Xiaoer tuchuang 小兒禿瘡

Take old soil from an earthen wall. Mix in egg whites and apply to the scalp. Repeat this every other day, and after five days the condition will be cured.

Yong duonian chengtu, jizituan tiao cha. Liang ri yi huan, wu tian quan hao.

用多年城土，雞子溥調搽。兩日一換，五天全好。

Head scabs are medically called favus of the scalp and are similar to ringworm (*xian* 癬). Here is my guess about why this preparation was put together and why it worked: Presumably soil taken from inside an earthen wall had not been used to grow plants in a long while and so would not contain any microbes or unknown living plants. Eggs were used in classical Chinese medicine to cure rashes (*banzhen* 斑疹) and other skin conditions. When the mixture was rubbed on the head, probably the granular dirt would help the scalp to exfoliate by rubbing away some of the infected skin. Modern medicine tells us that eggs are a good source of vitamin B3, and one of the signs of vitamin B3 deficiency is a skin rash.

It seems that 99.9% of the atoms in the human body contain sodium, potassium, calcium, magnesium, phosphorous, sulfur, and chlorine, which all have soil as their major source. These chemicals are necessary for growth. Favus was widespread throughout the world before the advent of modern therapies. The illustrious composer of Western classical music George Frederick Handel (1685–1759) had his head shaved to prevent scalp infections and, as was the custom at the time, wore a wig in public.

P62b. Many Years of Frostbite
Duonian dongchuang 多年凍瘡

Use eggplant, brushwood, wild pepper. Prepare by boiling them well in clean water. Wash the skin suffering from frostbite and it will heal.

Yong qie, chai, huajiao, aoshui xiz hi, zi hao.

用茄、柴、花椒，熬水洗之，自好。

For people who spent long periods of time outdoors in winter, especially in the freezing temperatures of north and northeast China, and when they do not have adequate clothing, frostbite was a recurring problem. Analyzed from the traditional Chinese point of view, frostbite is presented as restricted circulation, lack of *qi* 氣 and blood (*xue* 血) because of excessive exposure to extreme cold. The affected area becomes pale or purple, with numbness and an itchy pain. The condition becomes one of *qi* deficiency (*qixu* 氣虛), blood stasis (*xueyu* 血瘀), and dampness (*shi* 濕) which means watery and swelling, possibly infection characterized by excess pain and redness.

Besides warming the affected areas, treatment included decoctions, or salves placed on the affected areas. From the recipe given in this manual, it is unclear how to apply these boiled plant items. The boiling would have removed some toxins from the herbs and they could have been mixed with a substance such as animal fat allowing the mixture to be rubbed on as a salve or ointment (*gao* 膏), or covered in a cloth and called a poultice (*gaoyao* 膏藥).

P62c. Flavored Ginseng/Herbal Soup
Jiawei xionggui tang 加味芎歸湯

It Always Works. One *liang* of *angelica sinesis*, seven *qian* of Sichuan lovage root, a tortoise shell about the size of a hand that has been ground to powder and baked with vinegar, add woman's hair formed into a ball and baked in a lump of clay the size of an egg. Boil these four tastes in a pan with two cups of water. When served in a large bowl it will clear the five senses and [the patient will] feel as if being born again. Whether the birth was live or stillborn, joints are stiff, the effect [relief] will be as if from the gods.

Baishi baiyan. Danggui yi liang, Chuanxiong qi qian, guiban shou da yi pian cu zhi yanmo, furen toufa ru jizituan da yi gu, watu bei cun xing. Yishang si wei he yi, shui er wan, jian yi da wan fu. Ru ren xing wu li ji sheng. Huo taisi, huo jiaogu bu kaiyong, fu ci fang, qi xiao ru shen.

百試百驗。當歸一兩，川芎七个，龜板手大一片醋炙研末，婦人頭髮如雞子溥大一固，瓦土焙存性。以上四味合一，水二碗，煎一大碗服。如人行五里即生。或胎死，或交骨不開用，服此方，其效如神。

This seems to be an all-purpose preparation, much like chicken soup is recommended for general relief from malaise in Western countries. It was a pain reliever and a muscle relaxant, and may have most often been prescribed for general pain and low energy. *Angelica sinensis* is written as *danggui* 當歸 in this manual. It is a type of ginseng indigenous to East Asia that grows in the cool high-altitude mountainous regions of China, Korea, and Japan and is sometimes called "female ginseng." The yellowish-brown root is harvested in the fall. It has blood-thinning effects and can affect the muscles of the uterus, referenced here in the mention of a condition caused by childbirth. See S. Y. Goh and K. C. Loh, "Gynaecomastia and the Herbal Tonic Dong Quai," *Singapore Medical Journal* 42.3 (2001): 115–116, PMID: 11405562. Sichuan lovage root is a Western medical name for *chuanxiong* 川芎, a flowering plant in the carrot family and widely used in Chinese herbal recipes. Its Latin name is *ligusticum striatum*. It helps to relieve painful swelling of the joints.

Tortoise shells have many healthy medical effects, among them to nourish the liver and kidneys, to strengthen tendons and bones. The purpose of the woman's hair baked in a lump of mud was probably to extract the chemicals and nutrients from both the hair and the mud. The condition of one's hair is determined by the kidney (*shen* 腎). A healthy kidney free of stress will produce healthy hair which contains the vital energy (*jing* 精) produced by the kidney system. The resulting liquid mixture could be flavored by adding any of the four tastes: sweet (*tian* 甜), salty (*xian* 鹹), sour (*suan* 酸), or bitter (*ku* 苦).

The body was in a general weakened condition and the blood needed nourishing. The *chuanxiong* 川芎 flowering plant in the carrot family was often prescribed to reinvigorate the body's systems. An example to heal a body that has suffered a trauma is in Bao Xiangao 鮑相璈, *Raising the Dead and Returning Life: Emergency Medicine of the Qing Dynasty* (*Qisi huisheng* 起死回生), trans. Lorraine Wilcox (Portland, OR: Chinese Medical Database, 2012), pp. 116–117.

小兒禿瘡　用多年城土雞子清調搽兩日一換五天
全好

多年凍瘡　用茄柴花微熬水洗之自好
百試
百驗

加味芎歸湯

當歸一兩　川芎七　龜板醋炙研末入頭髮
手六一片
個
如雞子清六一個
凡上焙存性
以上四味合一水二碗煎
大碗服如人行五里
即生或胎死或交骨不開用
服此方其效如神

P63a. No Breast Milk [Lactation] Following Childbirth
Chanhou wunai 產後無奶

Use three *qian* of lettuce leaves. Roast and grind them. Drink them with yellow rice wine. The milk will then flow.

Yong wojucaizi san qian, chao yanmo. Huangjiu song xia, nai ji xia.

用萵苣菜子三个，炒研末。黃酒送下，奶即下。

In this case following childbirth the new mother is exhausted and feels weak and sore. After the baby is born, some of the mother's blood will be converted into breast milk which results in a deficiency in blood (*xuexu* 血虛) and energy (*qixu* 氣虛), both of which are needed to produce milk. It is normal for new mothers to feel weak after childbirth. Preparing herbal decoctions during the confinement period helps the body address the deficiencies.

Stagnation of the breast milk, poor lactation, means the milk is not moving down the ducts and out of the nipple, causing poor milk flow. This deficiency or stagnation of *qi* 氣 can lead to breast fullness, distension, pain, and engorgement. Likewise, the muscles of the uterus are in a somewhat painful condition immediately following birth.

During the time of recovery from a livebirth or a stillbirth, the chemical changes in the body produce combinations of strong emotions. These emotions of stress, anger, resentment, frustration, and often depression are the main causes of the physical blockages that reduce the production or flow of breast milk and impede recovery of the uterine muscles. Lettuce, as recommended in this prescription, is known for its ability to regulate *qi* circulation and calm the spirit. It also helps to clear heat, resolve dampness, and regulate water circulation.

P63b. The Meridians Are Blocked
Jingmai butiao 經脈不調

Take three *qian* of leaves from both a safflower and a boneset plant. Grind them to powder and drink with yellow rice wine.

Yong honghua zelanye ge san qian, yanmo, huangjiu song xia.

用紅花、澤蘭葉各三个，研末，黃酒送下。

Three *qian* 錢 are equal to 11.19 grams or 0.39 ounce from each tree. Meridians (*jingmai* 經脈) are sometimes translated into English as channels (*jingluo* 經絡), which the Chinese distinguish as two different systems within the body: channels for blood, meridians for energy. But in my translations in this manual, the separation of the two is usually not distinguished. See my note in P3.

As used in this translation, meridians are the pathways of energy (*qi* 氣) and blood (*xue* 血) that flow continually through the body. Any disruption of this flow because of constriction, injury, or illness, causes an unbalance within the body, always leading to negative effects. The negative effects can be anything from a tumor or a stroke to general lethargy. Safflower (*honghua* 紅花) is a plant. The flower and oil from the seeds are used as medicine to treat conditions such as high cholesterol, heart disease, stroke, and diabetes. Boneset (*zelan* 澤蘭) is a plant in the aster family. Its dried leaf and flowers are used as medicinal cures for influenza, the common cold, and symptoms of lung infections. Some of its chemicals might have mild activity against bacteria.

P63c. A Good Method for Washing the Eyes
Xiyan liangfang 洗眼良方

Evergreen roots with blue vitriol and green salt, these three [ingredients]. Buy ten portions. Boil and stir-fry them to get a strong fragrance. Use this to wash the eyes.

Kushen, danfan, qingyan san yang. Mai shi ge qian de. Zhao chao guo aogun, lian xin. Dai xi.

苦參、胆凡、青鹽三樣。買十个个的。着炒鍋熬滾，連馨。代洗。

Evergreen roots can be called *kushen* 苦參. This is a slow-growing shrub also known as the sophora root, with the generic name of *radix sophorae flavescentis.*

Blue vitriol is a form of copper (II) sulfate. It works against pesticides, but modern medicine considers it an irritant to the eye that can cause inflammation to eyelids and clouding of the cornea. It is properly written *danfan* 胆矾 / 膽礬 (chalcanthite), but in this manual the second character has been simplified to *fan* 凡. When green salt (*qingyan* 青鹽) is called Magnus's green salt it refers to a variety named after the German scientist who reported the compound in the 1830s, which was an inorganic compound not soluble in water. But we can assume the salt recommended in this medical recipe was a soluble variety. This is properly called halite or halide mineral salt, commonly known as rock salt, which is the mineral form of sodium chloride.

When these two ingredients, chalcanthite and halite, are used together, the effect is heat clearing (*qingre* 清熱) and detoxifying (*jiedu* 解毒).

Inflammation of the eyelid was caused by wind heat (*fengre* 風熱). Itchy eyelids are termed allergic conjunctivitis. Symptoms can include reddening, tearing, soreness, even burning or painful sensations. When the condition appears in the fall or spring, seasonal allergic conjunctivitis is diagnosed. Classical Chinese medicine concludes that particular internal organs are not giving enough nourishment (*yang* 養) to the eyes, which rely on the essence (*jing* 精) of the organs for their nourishment. Various parts of the eye and eyelid are correlated to particular organs.

P63d. Constipation in a Child
Xiaoer piji 小兒痞積

One *jin* of walnut meat, four *liang* of tannic acid, boiled together. Add four *liang* of honey. You can take this medicine at any time.

Hetaoren yi jin, pishao si liang, tong zhu. Rumi si liang. Buju shi zhan [fu?].

核桃仁一斤，皮硝四兩，同煮。入蜜四兩。不拘時貼 [服 ？]。

As used when this manual was produced, one *jin* 斤 was 570 grams or 1.316 pounds. The *liang* 兩 was 37.301 grams or 1.316 ounces. The *qian* 錢 (dividing the *liang* by 10) was 3.7301 grams or 0.1316 ounce. Tannic acid such as the *pixiao* 皮硝 mentioned here is often used in classical Chinese medicine to treat intestinal disorders, such as diarrhea and dysentery, constipation, and intestinal parasites. The *pixiao* are types of fungi called mirabilites, classified as "purgative herbs that drain downward," and their main purpose is to treat constipation. They are called purgative because they remove excess heat in the intestines and/or stomach. They are said to be cold in nature in order to cool heat. Mirabilite is also known as Glauber's salt. It is a hydrous sodium sulfate mineral with the chemical formula $Na_2SO_4 \cdot 10H_2O$. It is found around saline springs.

Bitter ingredients like mirabilites have a cleansing action on the body that clears heat and promotes elimination via urination or bowel movements. But tannins are very astringent, causing a puckering feeling in the mouth, which is why this recipe calls for a generous amount of honey to be added to the mixture.

Note that the final Chinese character in this recipe, *zhan* 貼, must be incorrect, because it means "a tasteless broth." In another version of this manual that I consulted the final character was *dan* 胆, meaning gallbladder. The word *dan* if written in its complete form is 膽. The person who wrote out the text for the woodblocks for P61 to P64 (or the person who cut the blocks) used several simplified styles of writing characters. If we simplify the right-hand phonetic signifier of the character *zhan* 詹, it is simplified as *zhan* 占. This is the word combined with the semantic signifier (the radical) for internal organs (*rou* 月) as written in my version. My colleague Dr. Stone Chen, however, feels the word was mistaken on both my version and the other version of this manual I consulted, and the word should have been *fu* 服, so the final phrase should be *bujushi fu* 不拘時服, meaning you can take the medicine at any time.

P63e. Inadvertently Swallowed Copper and Iron [Metals]
Wutun tongtie 悮吞銅鐵

Use bones from a sheep which are burned to ashes and ground up into two portions. Place this in rice gruel and drink it down. The metal will be excreted.

Yong yangjinggu, shaohui yanmo er qian. Mitang song xia, ji chu.

用羊脛骨，燒灰研末二个。米湯送下，即出。

As if we needed proof, this old medical recipe tells us that children (because this problem follows the previous one about constipation in a child) have long liked to put things into their mouth (in this case some metal objects). It might have been small round copper coins in common use for centuries in China, round with a square hole in the middle, were strung together, leading to the idea of strings of cash (*yi diaoqian* 一弔錢).

The gruel recommended here would promote a natural bowel movement. Many people in East Asia like to drink a calming warm rice gruel (*zhou* 粥) when they feel under the weather, so the child or person who swallowed the metal would take it as a natural preparation to help them feel better. A soup or gruel made with bones is a nutrient-rich and easily digested medicine for everyday health. The broth produced from ground animal bones is a mineral-rich strengthening food for healing support during recovery of an illness or surgery.

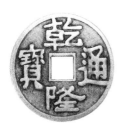

A traditional Chinese coin called "cash" (*qian* 錢) from the Qianlong Period (1736–1795)

Sheep bones were likely to be available in most parts of China. But why sheep bones? Research has shown many beneficial effects of sheep bones. See Keguang Han et al., "Effects of Lactobacillus Helveticas Fermentation, on the Ca^{2+} Release and Antioxidative Properties of Sheep Bone Hydrolysate," *Korean Journal for Food Science of Animal Resources* 38.6 (December 2018): 1144–1154, DOI: 10.5851/kosfa.2018.e32. Then again, perhaps recommending sheep bones is in the tradition of sympathetic medicine, since sheep droppings are small and discrete, somewhat like the expulsion of a coin would be.

P63f. Painful Swelling from a Scorpion Sting
Xiezhe zhongteng 蠍蜇腫疼

Use a piece of blue vitriol and rub it on the affected area. To have the pain disappear, immediately dab on cold water.

Danfan yi kuai cha huanchu, lishi zhiteng, yong liangshui cha.

胆凡一塊搽患處，立時止疼，用涼水搽。

We assume the characters written here as *danfan* 胆凡 should correctly be written as *danfan* 胆矾 / 膽礬, meaning chalcanthite, or blue vitriol which is a form of copper (II) sulfate (also mentioned in P63c). Copper sulfate has been used in many parts of the world as an antiseptic and for pain relief. It is classified as an irritant and is highly toxic, so only small doses should be used, but they are very effective. Scorpion stings are also mentioned in P52.

In stinging a person, the scorpion injects a venom into its victim. The venom contains a complex mix of toxins that affect the nervous system (neurotoxins). This can cause severe upper abdominal pain associated with nausea and vomiting. There is often swelling of the skin. There can be a rapid increase in blood pressure with sweating. Applying cold water would have an immediate, positive effect. Children can have a severe reaction to a scorpion sting and exhibit inconsolable crying.

産後無奶　經脉不調　洗眼良方　小兒痞積　悞吞銅鐵　蝎蜥腫疼

産後無奶
即下　用商苜菜子三十个炒研末黄酒送下

經脉不調
下　用紅花澤蘭藥各三十研末黄酒送下

洗眼良方
苦參胆凡青盬三樣買十个个的着炒
鍋整滾連礬代洗

小兒痞積
核桃仁一斤炭硝四兩同煮入蜜四兩
不拘時貼

悞吞銅鐵
用羊脛骨烧灰研末一个米湯送下即
下云

蝎蜥腫疼
朋几一塊搽患處立時止疼用涼水搓

P64a. Worms Have Entered the Ear
Zhuchong ruer 諸蟲入耳

Use some cat urine, not more than seven portions. The worms will come out. The way to get cat urine: Let the cat smell garlic and the cat will pee.

Yong maoniao xie xu man qi, ji chu. Qu maoniao fa: Yong suan mo maobi, ji you.

用貓尿些湏滿七，即出。取貓尿法：用蒜抹貓鼻，即有。

The word for worms (*chong* 蟲) could also mean insects. The assumption here is that some sort of insect has entered the ear canal where it is causing discomfort or irritation. Modern doctors might term this a parasitic invasion, but the wisdom of the therapy prescribed here is that an actual bug, a fly or a worm, is causing the distress. By inserting a liquid that will offend the insect, it will come out of the ear.

The therapy further assumes a connection between urine and garlic. Raw garlic has been used in various cultures as an herbal antibiotic to treat urinary tract infections. It is a staple in the pharmacopeia of classical Chinese medicine. In fact, garlic is considered to be one of the most widely used herbs in three of the world's major traditional health systems: Ayurvedic medicine that originated in India, classical Chinese medicine, and traditional European medicine. It is used for cleansing the body of pathogens. Apparently it will somewhat offend the cat, or at least shock it into emptying its bladder.

P64b. Deafness for Many Years
Duonian erlong 多年耳聾

Use the plant called *tianma* and grind it. Wrap it in a scrap of paper. Place this in the ear.

Yong tianmazi yansui. Zhi bao ru juzi yang. Qianru er nei.

用天麻子研碎。紙包如鋸子樣。嵌入耳內。

The generic name for *tianma* 天麻 is *gastrodia elata*. This is a tubular plant of the orchard family which grows upright and is fairly tall. It is used in classical Chinese medicine for calming the liver as well as for treating headaches, dizziness, tinnitus, and epilepsy. It is said to protect and calm neural networks, so recent interest has been shown in its possible treatment benefits in preventing and treating common neurological and metabolic disorders such as Alzheimer's, Parkinson's, Huntington's, epilepsy, liver disease, diabetes, and neuropathy.

The prescription is to be wrapped in a scrap of paper, no doubt wrinkled up into a small ball then placed in the ear but not intended to go deeply into the ear canal. In contemporary Western medicine, tinnitus (a ringing in the ear) has no effective cure.

P64c. Poor Eyesight
Que mengyan fang 雀矇眼方

A slice of the fresh liver from a lamb, fried in a pan. Burn it to a crisp, then eat it, that will be effective.

Qingyanggan yi jin, yu guo nei chao. Xian xun hou chi, ji hao.

青羊肝一斤，於鍋內炒。先熏後吃，即好。

Liver is in general considered a healthy meat. Sheep's liver is said to have properties of being both sweet and bitter, and it has a cooling (*liang* 涼) effect on the internal organs. It can tonify (nourish, *bu* 補) blood.

Animal liver, especially from beef or chicken, contains large amounts of vitamin A which is important for improving eyesight. Vitamin A, when combined with other antioxidants like zeaxanthin and lutein, plays a role in decreasing the risk of developing age-related eye health issues connected with eyesight. It promotes good vision in low light to improve night vision, the condition making it difficult to see clearly in dim light. Vitamin A helps to form an effective barrier to bacteria and viruses, reducing the risk of eye infections and is essential for maintaining photoreceptors, the special cells in the eye's retina that convert light into signals sent to the brain.

P64d. Gynecological Inflammation
Furen xiapan 婦人下瘤

Stamen of lotus, pomegranate rind, hornet's nest. Simmer in water, wash the affected area.

Lianxu, shiliupi, mapengwo jianshui, xi zhi.

連鬚、石榴皮、馬棚窩煎水，洗之。

Some of the Chinese characters used in this medical recipe as they appear in the manual are no longer in general use. Perhaps this is because the prescription deals with a somewhat delicate topic? In my copy of the manual, the character referring to "inflammation" *pan* 瘤 is written with the illness radical, officially pronounced *chuang* or *ne* but colloquially referred to as *bing* 疒, plus the inner portion that gives a phonetic indication of the pronunciation of the character *pan* 番, making up the full character *pan* 瘤. This character does not appear in many modern dictionaries or on much current software. The meaning could be disease or therapy (*fan* 翻) which is used in this manual. Concerning the characters for lotus stamen (*lianxu* 蓮鬚), in this manual the word for "lotus" is written as *lian* 連 without the radical for grass (*cao* 艸) that should be placed at the top of the character. The word for stamen (*xu* 鬚) is written as *xu* 須 in simplified Chinese.

As for the recipe itself: The stamen of lotus (*lianxu* 蓮須) has a sharp sweet taste. It has the functions of clearing the heart, benefiting the kidneys and an astringent essence. The pomegranate rind (*shiliupi* 石榴皮) is considered warm and sour. It can be used for patients with chronic diarrhea, bloody stool, anal prolapse, and abdominal pain.

The hornet's nest (*mapengwo* 馬棚窩) is often used in classical Chinese medicine. It has the functions of clearing away heat and toxins, dispelling wind and dredging collaterals, attacking toxins and treating sores, providing a warming (*yang* 陽) essence and benefiting the kidneys (*shen* 腎). I learned that in the Shandong 山東 dialect, the hornet's nest is pronounced as *mafengwo* 馬蜂窩. All of these ingredients are simmered in water which is then used to wash the affected area.

P64e. Exhausted/Anemic Blood
Zhengxuelao zheng 症血勞症

Root of a red peony, almond, burn to ashes. With yellow rice wine, drink it down.

Guiwei chishao, xingren, daodi hui. Huangjiu song xia.

歸尾赤芍、杏仁，到底灰。黃酒送下。

Anemia occurs in humans when the blood is low in red cells or hemoglobin, resulting in paleness or weakness. In classical Chinese medicine red peony roots are plants in the category that invigorate the blood (*huoxue* 活血). This means there is a lack of blood movement and this herb encourages blood flow. Ren peony clears heat (*qingre* 清熱), cools the blood (*liangxue* 涼血), clears liver fire (*ganre* 肝熱), and dispels blood stasis (*quxuezhi* 祛血滯). All of these actions benefit coronary health by promoting normal circulation, which is vital to maintaining a balance of *yin* 陰 and *yang* 陽. Modern doctors have found that peony contains a compound called paeoniflorin, which acts to calm the nerves and reduce the incidence of muscle spasms.

Almonds are known for the ability to strengthen (*bu* 補) two basic and crucial aspects of the body's health and functioning: the vital *qi* 氣 that gives energy to the system, and the strength of purpose and resolve (*jing* 精) which the human psyche gives to this process. Almonds have a laxative effect, which works to assist blood flow through the system.

P64f. Treating Tuberculosis Swellings
Zhi qiluochuang 治氣瘰瘡

Raw rhubarb, Chinese ground orchid, the underground stem shoots of a radish. A small portion of each ground up. [Immerse in] milk and daub it on.

Shengdahuang, baiji, shuiluoshougen. Ge dengfen, wei mo. Ruzhi, tiao cha.

生大黃、白芨、水羅首根。各等分，為末。乳汁，調搽。

The three basic ingredients are raw rhubarb (*shengdahuang* 生大黃), Chinese ground orchid (*baiji* 白芨), and roots of a radish (*shuiluoshougen* 水羅首根). The word radish is usually written as *luobo* 蘿蔔, and the roots of a radish would be written *shuiluobogen* 水蘿蔔根. The radish is used as a Chinese medicine that can treat lung-related symptoms, such as phlegm and cough.

The condition named here as tuberculosis swellings (*qiluochuang* 氣瘰瘡) is commonly referred to in Western medicine as scrofula, and has the medical name of "cervical tuberculous lymphadenitis." Because of breathing in air that is contaminated with mycobacterium bacteria, the bacteria irritates and inflames the lymph nodes in the neck, causing swelling to occur. The swelling can be painful, and in some cases the swelling refuses to heal. The swelling has been regularly linked to tuberculosis so there is a high risk that a person with the condition is contagious. A brief description of a patient with this condition is given in A. K. Pannu and S. Pannu, "Scrofula," *QJM: An International Journal of Medicine* 110.8 (August 2017): 535, DOI: 10.1093/qjmed/hcx098, accessed June 10, 2021.

The condition was probably not uncommon in the market towns and cities of China in the 1860s when foundries and light industry was spreading and when coal and other ores were taken from the ground and were in demand for the manufacture of products. If there was a rail line in the area, the steam engines always spilled out coal smoke, ashes, and fumes. Today's world is noted for air that is polluted with irritants of all types. This medical condition continues to be of concern to public health officials in many countries.

諸蟲入耳　用猫尿此滴齒七即止取猫尿法用薤
鼻即有

多年耳聾　用天麻子研碎紙包如疤子樣次入耳內

雀矇眼方　青羊肝一斤於鍋內炒先重後哈即好

婦人下瘤　連鬍石榴皮馬桐罵前水洗之

症血勞症　歸尾赤勺杏仁到底灰黃酒送下

治氣瘰瘡　生大黃白芨水羅首根各等分為末乳汁
調搽

Appendix A

PUBLICATION HISTORY OF THE *SEVENTY-TWO THERAPIES*

The book translated here is a collection of herbal recipes for treating a variety of medical conditions. They are simple remedies meant to be offered in emergency situations when quick relief was needed because the patient was in distress.

The translation in this book is from the woodblock edition I bought in June 2013 in Beijing. Its front cover was missing, and that would have had the title, name of the publisher, and a date of publication. As I began to research similar works in Chinese, I concluded that this was a version of the collection known as the *Seventy-Two Therapies* (*Qishier fanzheng* 七十二翻症). I drew this conclusion even though my woodblock copy has thirty-seven folio pages, allowing for seventy-four illustrated recipes and its final two folio pages 38 and 39 have twenty-one recipes listed and described but not illustrated. My copy also has some pages missing from the numbered folio pages, and places where at least three half pages have been torn out. In other words, my copy originally contained over eighty-one therapies.

The designation of *Seventy-Two Therapies* has been the generally accepted title for this collection of herbal medical recipes. Various publishers in China from the mid-Qing 清 period (my copy likely dates from the 1860s) on began to issue editions of this collection. They re-cut the woodblocks with its illustrations and text, put their imprint on the collection, and sold it to the public. As they did so, they often made variations on its basic title. Some of the variations in the title were: *Elaborations on the Seventy-Two Therapies* (*Xiuxiang qishier fanzheng* 繡像七十二翻症); *Seventy-Two Therapies: Illustrated* (*Qishier fanzheng quantu* 七十二翻症全圖); *Seventy-Two Therapies: Illustrated and Explained* (*Qishier fan tushuo* 七十二翻圖説). These are just some of the examples; more are given in the text below.

My search to discover the publication history of this title in China was conducted largely online. The internet is a wonderful galaxy of information and images. As we all know, it sometimes beams light at us, and sometimes it twinkles, and regularly it fades from view leaving emptiness in its place. A number of sites I located in my search had photos of a complete set of medical remedies by showing every page of the item in their collection. Others showed a few pages, some only presented the title page with publication information and a few of the earliest pages. The sites that had complete copies allowed me to compare individual prescriptions among the various copies, as well as to note the style of the drawing and the type of clothing the illustrated patients wore which gives some indication of when the drawings were prepared, and the order in which the prescriptions were presented. When I realized that the same set of prescriptions appeared in differing sequences in various publications, I concluded that the prescriptions did not have a fixed sequential order. My reactions to these and related points appear in the comments below.

Through online searching I found references to quite a few of the woodblock editions that were issued. In the period of the Republic (*Minguo* 民國, 1911–1949) publishers began to reprint the earlier woodblock editions by using lithography (*shiyin* 石印) printing. In this process an image of the page with its illustrations and text was put on a metal plate; through inking and pressing on the plate, copies were produced. This made it even easier to reprint a book, because it only required an image of the original pages from the book that was obtained by the book pirates. It was no longer necessary to cut a new set of woodblocks. Without copyright conventions or laws in place, the purpose of copying and printing the book was only to make money, and the publishers who did this were in the category of what we term "book pirates." The new publisher could then use the images to reprint it as a pirated edition, which had not been authorized by the holder of the original carved woodblocks. The new publisher used the name of their own publishing company. By 1916 several publishers in China began selling their own editions of this collection of medical recipes. Sometimes they only removed the name of the original publisher and inserted their own company name. It is possible that in some cases they allowed the name of the original publisher to remain, because all they wanted was the income from the copies they sold in the marketplace, and the reputation or prestige of their own brand was not of special interest to them.

Today online sites principally in mainland China and Taiwan offer versions of this collection produced by woodblock printing, lithography, and even a few hand-drawn copies are for sale to the public. I tried to discover how many versions of this collection issued under different titles have been produced. The information below lists the information I found, doing the bulk of my online research in 2021 and 2022. I did a quick online check of these sites in late 2023 to find that a number of the commercial sites were still open with copies of the individual pages still available to see.

At present many of the available copies of this title in woodblock, lithographic reprints, or in hand-written versions, can be found on online sites in mainland China and Taiwan that offer old books for sale. As of 2023, a large number were concentrated on the site of the Confucius Used Book Store (*Kongfuzi jiushudian* 孔夫子舊書店) or the Confucius Net (*Kongfuzi wang* 孔夫子網, Kongfz.com). Many other sites act as marketing centers (much like Amazon.com). They list book titles they will supply which are on sale by other vendors. Some of these marketing sites are:

(1) 360doc.com is a China site for information about many things, advertising itself as the "individual's library" (*geren tushuguan* 個人圖書館).

(2) Qudiandi.com 點滴拍賣 is a B2C (business to customer) online auction marketplace specializing in old books, antiques, etc. It is in Beijing and seems to be a legitimate online platform. It claims that it is registered with the government. It seems to be similar to Amazon.com marketplace.

(3) Ruten.com.tw 露天網 is a company called Open Air Daily International Information Co., Ltd. (*Lutian shiji guoji zixun gufen youxiangongsi* 露天市集國際資訊股份有限公司). It is an online marketplace in Taiwan that looks exactly like Amazon.com.

(4) Wantubizhi.com 萬圖壁紙, meaning Ten Thousand Wallpapers, is a computer desktop wallpaper website in Taiwan listing all sorts of things.

(5) The site 7788.com identifies itself as a commercial market (*shangcheng* 商城).

Several photos of pages of different editions were available online, some of them taken from other sites or from one of the Kongfuzi sites. Not all of the listings on the various sites provide detailed publication information, and not all of the sites reproduced all of the pages. From the online listings of this work available during my searches, I have tried to give a sense of the various editions of this title that were created.

An interesting discussion of a number of the editions and comments about this title by Lai Baishan 萊白山 posted on January 17, 2015 were found on https://www.360doc.com/content/15/0117/11/762362_441511002.shtml, accessed January 2022, and November 20, 2023.

These sites can change their content at will. Sometimes the listing with illustrations of all the pages is left on the site by a seller even after the item has been sold. These became useful records for me when I found them. Some sites gave the size of the volume, or the city where the copy was located. The descriptions accompanying the online listing rarely contained extensive commentary about the title, just enough basic details to allow a purchaser to make a decision about buying the item. Where available, below I have given some background information on the publishing houses that issued the editions in question. Also, when available based on online searching, I have listed some other titles put out by the company as a way of judging their general publishing program.

As mentioned above, on some of the online sites, all the pages of the title were posted. That allowed me to compare the medical recipes with those listed in my personal woodblock copy, which I used as the basis for the translations and illustrations in this book. The printed copies I examined were very similar to my own copy in several ways: The names of the therapies (label), the description of the presenting symptoms, and the treatments prescribed were usually word-for-word the same. There were a few cases where the wording of a medical prescription differed, but those differences usually consisted only of a word or two. In a few cases it seems the woodblock carvers of my edition carved a wrong character. Most likely they were only following the words and style as written on the paper template pasted over the woodblock as their guide. (An illustrator would write a paper copy of the illustration and text to be carved into the woodblock. This was turned with the reverse side up and pasted on the woodblock, allowing the carvers to produce a cutting that would print with the "right side up," just as it was drawn.) Cases of incorrect or variant characters are pointed out in my comments on each recipe when they occur.

There were, however, two notable differences between my copy and the woodblock or lithographed copies I found online. First, the order in which the therapies were given varied in the different editions. This is explained in my Introduction as resulting from having new woodblocks cut in a different

order, with two therapies on each woodblock face. Carving the medical recipes in differing orders was unintentional and did not result in any difficulty
because the therapy label (the name assigned to the affliction), the presenting
symptoms, and the accompanying medical prescription remained the same.
The therapies never seem to have had a sequential numbering. Thus, even
after new woodblocks were cut or lithographic plates were copied, they could
be compiled and published in different sequences.

A second difference in the available versions are the style of the illustrations. Most of those available on the internet have distinct illustrations made
by a professional artist. The illustrations consist of a drawing of a patient in
distress, and usually an animal or insect representing the label of the affliction. In the Qing period males were required to wear their hair in the Manchu
style, shaving the forehead and keeping a long, plaited queue (*bianzi* 辮子, pig-
tail, braid). By 1916 this was no longer a required hairstyle and most males in
China began to grow their hair in the "contemporary" style of medium length
and combed. The changes in hairstyle were reflected in the new illustrations
prepared for post-Qing editions. One also sees that the people illustrated in
the 1916 versions no longer wear Qing-style robes, but instead sometimes have
Western-style trousers, though the patients in all the editions have informal
and loose-fitting clothing. Further, the illustrations in my copy are of a somewhat abstract and impressionistic style, which is discussed in my Introduction. It was those illustrations that helped me determine the probable date
of my copy as being from the 1860s. Most illustrations from the 1916 editions
onward gave more detailed and correctly proportioned images of the human
body. The majority of illustrations are of males, with only a few that seem they
could represent female bodies. The prescriptions that deal with women and
children were grouped in my version, and in some of the other published versions, at the end of the collection and were presented without illustrations and
without the insect or animal reference common to most of the recipes.

Note that when searching for listings of this work, the *Seventy-Two Therapies* usually appears as part of the collection titled *Illustrated Acupuncture Made
Easy, Two Volumes; Appendix of Seventy-Two Therapies* (*Huitu zhenjiu yixue, shangxia juan; fu qishier fanzheng* 繪圖針灸易學，上下卷；附七十二翻症). The key
title words to use when searching are "*Huitu zhenjiu*" 繪圖針灸 . . . , because
this is the way the *Seventy-Two Therapies* are listed in libraries or when for sale.
One can also start an online search with the keywords for *Seventy-Two* (*Qishier*

七十二) . . . , because that collection was regularly issued as an appendix (*fu* 附) of the longer *Illustrated Acupuncture* title. For the *Seventy-Two* . . . title I usually give the date when I accessed the online site in the list below, but do not list access dates for other material obtained from the internet.

Credit for the collection of the *Acupuncture Made Easy* (*Zhenjiu yixue* 針灸易學) is given to Li Shouxian 李守先 (1735–1809). He was born in present day Henan province, Changge city, Chating village 河南省長葛市茶亭村. In 1786, at the age of 51 he began treating people using acupuncture techniques in conjunction with the herbal medicines usually employed, in response to a severe malaria epidemic at the time. His approach was effective in a great number of the cases he treated so he compiled his research, and in 1798 published his findings under the title of *Acupuncture Made Easy*. After Li's death several of his students, Wang Ting 王庭, Wan Shaofeng 萬少峰, Gao Xiao 高蕭, and Xu Chong 許沖, published a number of his medical prescriptions, including both herbal preparations and acupuncture, under the title of *Seventy-Two Therapies Illustrated* (*Qishier fan tu* 七十二翻圖) in 1847. That edition had a preface (*xu* 序) written in the spring of 1847 by Xu Tianxi 許天錫, a colleague who praised the diligence and humanity of Li Shouxian and his confidence in the medical techniques Li recommended. (Xu Tianxi shared the same name with a Ming Dynasty literati Xu Tianxi 許天錫 [1461–1508] who was from Fujian province 福建省, received the advanced *jinshi* 進士 degree and served as a government official between 1499 and 1505.)

In subsequent years, both of these works were published together as a set under the title typically presented as *Illustrated Acupuncture Made Easy, Two Volumes; Appendix of Seventy-Two Therapies* (*Huitu zhenjiu yixue, shangxia juan; fu qishier fanzheng* 繪圖針灸易學，上下卷；附七十二翻症).

Each time a new publisher cut woodblocks for this work, they altered the title in order to distinguish it as their own imprint. Among the variations on the basic title *Seventy-Two Therapies* (*Qishier fanzheng* 七十二翻症) seen in the list of editions below are to be found: *On Medical Therapies Illustrated* (*Fanzheng tukao* 翻症圖考); *Seventy-Two Therapies* (*Qishier fanzheng quantu* 七十二翻症全圖); *New Edition of Diseases Illustrated* (*Xinkan fan tukao* 新刊翻圖考); *Elaborations on Medical Therapies* (*Xiuxiang fanzheng* 繡像翻症); *Newly Expanded Elaborations on Seventy-Four Therapies* (*Xinzeng xiuxiang qishisi fanzheng* 新增繡像七十四翻症). The list can continue, but what it tells us is that some of the basic concepts of modern marketing were well in place in late-Qing China. Among them was to make everything appear to be new, elaborated, and expanded. This approach seems to respond to a basic human desire for something "new," even if it does not conform to the treasured idea in pre-modern China that the original versions of the past were always to be preferred. Western scholars of China have presumed that an overwhelming respect for the past was a widely held preference among the people of China, but perhaps it was only an opinion embraced by Chinese elite scholars?

Note that I have used the complete form of Chinese characters (also called sinographs), but PRC sites usually use the simplified version (*jiantizi* 簡體字, which would be written as 简体字). Note also that nineteenth-century China publishing houses often used the term *tang* 堂 (hall) in their business name. An example would be Sanyitang 三義堂 listed below. Since the early twentieth century, Chinese publishing companies often prefer to use *shuju* 書局. This term has been translated below as "book company," "bookstore," "publishing company," or "publishing house." An example would be *Guangyi shuju* 廣益書局, listed below as Guangyi Publishing House.

Qing Period Woodblock Editions

1798 Edition. From the year *Jiaqing san nian* 嘉慶三年, this was the *Acupuncture Made Easy* (*Zhenjiu yixue* 針灸易學) published by the author Li Shouxian. By tradition, later reprints of this title almost always included an Author's Preface (*zixu* 自序) written by Li Shouxian in 1798. I have not been able to see a woodblock copy of this edition.

1847 Edition. This is from the year *Daoguang ershiqi nian* 道光二十七年. I have seen this edition listed but have not been able to find a copy. Did this edition also include the newly prepared *Seventy-Two Therapies* (*Qishier fanzheng* 七十二翻症), or was that title initially issued as a separate publication?

1851 Edition. *Elaborations on the Seventy-Two Therapies* (*Xiuxiang qishier fanzheng* 繡像七十二翻症), published by Wenlintang 文林堂. According to the Korean site Kobay.co.kr, it was issued in *Xianfeng yuannian eryue* 咸豐元年二月 (February 1851). A photo of a portion of the title page that was on the site read *Elaborations on Medical Therapies* (*Xiuxiang fanzheng* 繡像翻症), "Newly Published Late Spring 1851" (*Xianfeng yuannian zhongchun xincheng* 咸豐元年仲春新成). This collection of medical recipes was originally compiled in 1847 but I have not found a copy, so this 1851 edition might be the first time the therapies were issued as a stand-alone title? Later in the 1800s it was usually added as an appendix (*fu* 附) to the titles of Li Shouxian's earlier work *Illustrated Acupuncture Made Easy* (*Huitu zhenjiu yixue* 繪圖針灸易學). The 1851 edition appeared for sale on the Korean Kobay site. The posting on the site is no longer available since it was removed in 2021 after the volume had been sold in 2019. A version of this edition that was obviously used by a medical practitioner who wrote many comments on pages in the book was on https://book.kongfz.com/7593/2584059799/, accessed January 11, 2022, and November 29, 2023. Some of the pages were shown on this site. The medical recipes shown were possibly to use for a decoction called Angelica and Notopterygium (*Danggui qianghuo tang* 當歸羌活湯) that could be used for stroke patients with heat (*re* 熱) symptoms, such as cough and excessive phlegm. This copy appeared to have the word Capital (*jingdu* 京都) written in the folded *fengbu* 縫部 section of the folio pages. Size is 7.95 inch (20.2 cm) h. × 5.12 inch (13 cm) w. It was located in Henan province, Zhengzhou 河南省鄭州市.

Wenlintang was an active publisher during the *Xianfeng* 咸豐 period (1851–1861). They were active in Guangdong province. They put out titles intended to be welcomed by the general public. Their titles seem to have been inexpensively produced and in some cases, based on an online photo of one of their editions, were woodblock prints showing many ink smudge marks. They issued books such as *The Four Books in Large Characters, Expanded Edition, Punctuated, with Side Notes* (*Dazi sishu zengbu quandian pangxun* 大字四書增補圈點旁訓), in two volumes; *Seven-Line Verse by a Thousand Poets* (*Qiyan qianjia shi* 七言千家詩); and the standard text for all learners, the *Three Character Classic* (*Sanzijing* 三字經) in an illustrated version.

1870 Edition. *Seventy-Two Therapies* (*Qishier fanzheng* 七十二翻症). Woodblocks of this title were cut and printed (*keban* 刻板) by Wannan Jingyuantang 宛南經元堂 (Wannan 宛南 is a place name, historically associated with Shanghai 上海 or Henan 河南), *Tongzhi jiunian* 同治九年. This edition was earlier printed and distributed in 1860 (*Gengjia shuayin guangchuan* 庚甲刷印廣傳). Some pages were illustrated. This copy was possibly from Fujian province, Xiamen city 福建省廈門市. See https://www.ruten.com.tw/item/show?21745312784790, accessed November 20, 2023. The 1870 edition was mentioned in https://www.360doc.com/content/15/0117/11/762362_441511002.shtml, accessed

November 29, 2023. Also on https://book.kongfz.com/252611/3636178052/, accessed December 4, 2023.

The Jingyuantang publishing house dates back at least to the early 1700s. Among the titles it issued that were located for sale online in 2022 were:

(1) *Annotations on the Genealogy of Surnames* (*Xingshi zupu jianzhi* 姓氏族譜箋釋), 8 volumes (*juan* 卷). By Xiong Junyun 熊峻運. Jingyuantang 經元堂, *Yongzhen er–san* 雍正二三 (1724–1725).

(2) *Complete Collection with Annotations and Summaries of The Four Books* (*Sishu shuzhu cuoyan daquan* 四書疏註撮言大全), 37 *juan*. Edited by Hu Feicai 胡斐才. Jingyuantang 經元堂, 1763.

(3) *The Butterfly Medium (Spirit)* (*Hudie mei* 蝴蝶媒). By Nanyue daoren 南嶽道人 (who was active in the eighteenth century). Four *juan*. Jingyuantang 經元堂, in print by 1754. Nanyue daoren translates as Daoist of the South Mountain, one of the five great mountains of China regarded as sacred by the Daoists. The mountain itself is Hengshan 衡山 in Hunan province 湖南省. The volumes are 9.3 inch (23.7 cm) h. × 5.4 inch (13.8 cm) w.

(4) *The Four Secrets* (*Simi quanshu* 四秘全書), Volume 12. By Yin Youben 尹有本. Jingyuantang 經元堂, *Jiaqing gengchen ershiwu* 嘉慶庚辰二十五 (1820).

(5) *Illustrated Encyclopedia for Daily Use* (*Huitu wanbao quanshu* 繪圖萬寶全書). Compiled by Chen Meigong 陳眉公 and Mao Huanwen 毛煥文. Jingyuantang 經元堂, *Jiaqing* 嘉慶 era (1796–1820) publication.

1874 Edition. *Elaborations on Medical Therapies* (*Xiuxiang fanzheng* 繡像翻症). Published as a woodblock edition by Jianyutang *keben* 鑒餘堂刻本. *Tongzhi shisan nian* 同治十三年 (1874). The book has 78 pages. Listed in *Dictionary of Chinese Medical Books* Compilation Committee (*Zhongguo yiji da cidian* 中國醫籍大辭典), ed. the *Dictionary of Chinese Medical Books* (*Bianzuan weiyuanhui* 編纂委員會), Shanghai Scientific Press (*Shanghai kexue jishu chubanshe* 上海科學技術出版社), 2002. Database: Shutongwen Ancient Books Database (*Shutongwen guji shujuku* 書同文古籍數據庫), Chinese Medicine Chinese Herbs Ancient Texts Third Section (*Zhongyi zhongyao guji daxi san bian* 中醫中藥古籍大系三編), https://guji.unihan.com.cn/Web#/book/ZYZYSB/page?pageId=MTQ2NDI1ODIzNzc%3DOA%3D%3D, accessed 2021. It appears to be no longer available as of November 29, 2023.

1886 Edition. The inside title page reads: *Elaborations on Medical Therapies* (*Xiuxiang fanzheng* 繡像翻症), Juyuantang 聚元堂, *Guangxu shier nian* 光緒

十二年 (1886). Size is 7.5 inch (19 cm) h. × 4.72 inch (12 cm) w. Listed by the seller as *Capital Edition, Newly Cut [Woodblocks] of Therapies Illustrated (Elaborations on Therapies)* (*Jingduben xinke fanzheng tukao [Xiuxiang fanzheng]* 京都本新刻翻症圖考[繡像翻症]). Located in Shanxi province, Jinzhong 山西省晉中市. Clearly a woodblock edition with ink smudge marks from the printing process. This is a volume where the words "Capital Edition" (*jingdu ben* 京都本) appear. https://book.kongfz.com/13412/830881321/, accessed July 28, 2021, and November 29, 2023.

In 1901 a trained doctor, Wang Jukui 王聚奎, opened a pharmacy in Luoyang named the Juyuantang. Wang both sold herbal medicines and practiced medicine. Wang came from a family of medical practitioners. His great grandfather, Wang Xuequan 王學權, had published the book *Essays from the Chongqing Hall* (*Chongqingtang suibi* 重慶堂隨筆) in 1808 that was also known as *Writings on Medicine* (*Yixue suibi* 醫學隨筆). His grandfather, Wang Shixiong 王士雄 (1808–1868), published many books on medical research. Among the ways of addressing the cholera epidemics plaguing China at the time, Wang Shixiong recommended ingesting the mung bean and garlic. He pointed out that a sanitary environment was crucial to decrease the cholera infection rate. He said greater bodily sterility could be maintained by eating fewer fats and sugars. He advocated for increased sanitation in all environments and suggested taking measures such as keeping rooms well ventilated and sanitary. He said burning Chinese rhubarb and capillary Artemisia would dramatically reduce outdoor contamination. He advocated purifying water to avoid cholera transmission by using alum and realgar. The contributions of Wang Shixiong have been studied by Yu Lin; see Lin Yu, "Wang Shixiong's Medicine Career," *Chinese Medicine and Culture* 3.4 (2020): 254–256, https://journals.lww.com/cmc/fulltext/2020/10000/wang_shixiong_s_medicine_career.11.aspx.

Coming from such a prominent medical family, Wang Jukui himself became an accomplished scholar, received the *jinshi* 進士 degree in 1874, and was appointed as an imperial physician because of his medical knowledge. When he opened his pharmacy the Juyuantang in 1901, because of his official appointment by the imperial court, he took as his sobriquet (*hao* 號) the words "Capital" (*jingdu* 京都). There seems to be no record of Wang or his pharmacy publishing medical information. But a number of the works listed in this Appendix contain the words *jingdu* on the folded (*fengbu* 縫部) or fishtail (*yuwei* 魚尾). The folded section is at the outer edges of the pages, where the single printed sheet was folded. The phrase was probably used to indicate the publication was "official" or "authorized," or in some ways "standard." For example, it appears on the 1851 edition listed above in this Appendix. The connection to Wang Jukui and his Juyuantang pharmacy which opened fifty years after the phrase Capital first appeared in 1851 is not certain.

A plaque used by the Juyuantang pharmacy is currently in the Luoyang Folk Museum. It reads: "Juyuantang deals in Chinese medicinal materials to treat various intractable diseases, focusing on the treatment of tics" (*Juyuantang jingying Zhongyaocai, zhiliao gezhong yinan zhazheng, zhongdian zhiliao choudong zheng* 聚元堂經營中藥材，治療各種疑難雜症，重點治療抽動症).

The family has continued to practice medicine. In the government-mandated business reorganization of 1954, the pharmacy was folded into a larger medical supply unit in Luoyang and the owners left the city to practice medicine elsewhere. In 1983 the pharmacy was re-established as an independent business. In 2000, Ms. Wang Wenli 王雯麗 became the seventh-generation successor of Juyuantang, which presently is located in Luoyang on Guansheng Street (*Guansheng jie* 關聖街) in front of the Guanlin Temple (*Guanlinmiao qian* 關林廟前) This is a temple dedicated to the deity Guangong 關公.

See https://www.easyatm.com.tw/wiki for "聚元堂," accessed December 24, 2021. No longer available as of November 29, 2023.

1886 Edition. *Seventy-Two Medical Therapies Completely Illustrated* (*Qishier fanzheng quantu* 七十二翻症全圖). Full publication information is not given. This appears to be a woodblock edition. This site gives a fully illustrated version. This has the word Capital (*jingdu* 京都) written in the fishtail (*yuwei* 魚尾) folded section (*fengbu* 縫部). Its size is 10.35 inch (26.3 cm) h. × 5.43 inch (13.8 cm) w. This appears to be the edition that was later reprinted in 1939 in a lithographed copy by the Xiaozhong Book Company (*Xiaozhong shuju* 曉鐘書局), and is listed below. The online site had illustrations for eighty-seven medical recipes taken from the publication. See https://www.qudiandi.com/product/item/pid/10061934.html, accessed August 2021, and November 29, 2023.

1889 Editions. The Sanyitang 三義堂 publishing house issued the *Seventy-Two Therapies*, probably as part of the larger text of *Acupuncture Made Easy*. It appears that other publishers later reprinted (pirated) this edition, giving it different titles but keeping in the attribution to the Sanyitang on the title page. Thus I found three copies of this work attributed to Sanyitang, each with a similar but different title, and a fourth attributed to the pu blisher Shenyu-tang 慎餘堂. It seems impossible to distinguish between the authentic Sanyi-tang version of this title and those of the pirated versions. These versions are listed separately below as 1889 editions.

Sanyi 三義 usually refers to the three historical figures who banded together to oppose injustice. Best known of these is Guan Yu 關羽, who is honored as the Daoist deity Guangong 關公. The other two were Liu Bei 劉備 and Zhang Fei 張飛. Among the characteristics they all shared was integrity (*yi* 義). Other characteristics ascribed to them were loyalty (*zhong* 忠), honesty (*xin* 信), and bravery (*yong* 勇). The phrase and the deity are recognized by most people affiliated with Chinese communities everywhere in the world. Guangong has become the patron deity of students, the military, businesses, treated as a protector, God of Wealth, and symbol of determination and principle.

Sanyitang as a publisher may have been active between 1875 and 1908. Several libraries in the United States hold copies of the Sanyitang imprint dated 1889. Among other titles with a publishing date of 1889 published by Sanyitang were:

(1) *Genealogical Tables of the Fan Family* (*Fanshi zongpu* 樊氏宗譜) in two volumes (*juan* 卷).

(2) *Genealogical Tables of the Chen Family from Xishan* (*Xishan Chenshi zongpu* 錫山陳氏宗譜), compiled by Chen Xueqing 陳學卿 in twenty *juan*. This may refer to the Xishan of Jiangsu province 江蘇省錫山市.

(3) *Edited and Annotated Four Books Convenient for Students* (*Jiaokan zengzhu Sishu bianmeng* 校刊增註四書便蒙), ed. Yu Changcheng 俞長城, Jiao Yuanxi 焦袁熹, and Dai Youqi 戴有祺. These contain the commentary on the *Four Books* provided by the eminent philosopher Zhu Xi 朱熹.

(4) *New Edition Well Illustrated of Yuan and Heng's Compendium of Equine Cures* (*Xinkan zuantu Yuan Heng liaomaji* 新刊纂圖元亨療馬集), by Ming Dynasty veterinarians Yu Ren 喻仁 and Yu Jie 喻杰 from Anhui province, in six *juan*. Originally published in 1608, the two veterinarians later published *The Snake Classic* (*She Jing* 蛇經). Snakes are reptiles very familiar to those engaged in agriculture. In addition, snakes were used for medicinal purposes. This title was also published by Sanyitang. The two brothers further published *Compendium of the Water Buffalo Classic* (*Tuxiang shuihuangniujing hebing daquan* 圖像水黃牛經合併大全), in two *juan*. This work dealt with water buffalos, one of the most important animals that could be owned by a farmer.

Currently in Taiwan there is a company called Sanyitang Sinopharm Group (*Sanyitang guoyao jituan* 三義堂國藥集團), founded in 1981. Among its services are medicines to improve the sexual stamina and enjoyment of adults. The company claims that one of its founders surnamed Zhang 張 prepared secret medical compounds for the imperial family in olden times for strengthening the kidney function and after continuous improvement, it has solved the afflictions of kidney deficiency, impotence, and premature ejaculation. It is unclear if there is a family connection to the historical Sanyitang publishing business, although as we see above, titles related to medical prescriptions were among the products of this publisher.

1889 Edition. *New Edition of Therapies Illustrated* (*Xinkan fan tukao* 新刊翻圖考). The inside cover reads *Elaborations on Therapies* (*Xiuxiang fanzheng* 繡像翻症), Sanyitang *zi* 三義堂梓. The character *zi* 梓 following the publisher's name indicates the publisher holds the actual woodblocks. Listed by the seller as *yichou nian* 已丑年 (1889). One volume. This is a woodblock edition. Size is listed as 8.27 inch (21 cm) h. × 4.72 inch (12 cm) w. https://www.ruten.com.tw/item/show?21849174211112, accessed July 28, 2021, and November 29, 2023.

1889 Edition. *Elaborations on Medical Therapies* (*Xiuxiang fanzheng* 繡像翻症). Published as a woodblock edition by Sanyitang 三義堂, *Guangxu shiwu nian* 光緒十五年 (1889). The edition is described as having an *Appendix of Seventy-Four Different Medical Therapies Illustrated* (*Futu miaohui qishisi zhong butong xingtai fanzheng* 附圖描繪七十四種不同形態翻症) but it is unclear if this was part of the printed title or was simply a continuation of the printed pages. Mentioned on http://www.360doc.com/content/15/0117/11/762362_441511002.shtml, accessed July 2021, and November 29, 2023. The book is listed in *Chinese Dictionary of Medical Books* (*Zhongguo yiji da cidian* 中國醫籍大辭典), ed. the Compilation Committee (*Bianzuan weiyuanhui* 編纂委員會). Shanghai Scientific Press (*Shanghai kexue jishu chubanshe* 上海科學技術出版社), 2002.

1889 Edition. *Therapies Illustrated; Appendix of Acupuncture for Cholera* (*Fanzheng tukao; fu huoluan zhenfa* 翻症圖考；附霍亂針法). Published by Sanyitang *kan* 三義堂刊, *Guangxu shiwu nian* 光緒十五年 (1889). Listed in Yan Shiyi 嚴世藝, ed., *Chinese Medical Books* (*Zhongguo yiji tongkao* 中國醫籍通考), Shanghai Zhongyixueyuan chubanshe 上海中醫學院出版社, 1990. See first edition, Vol. 3. Visible on some pages in the folded section (*fengbu* 縫部) is the word Capital (*jingdu* 京都). See https://www.ruten.com.tw/item/show?21835555105303, accessed July 28, 2021, and November 29, 2023. Several pages are illustrated. Clearly this is a woodblock edition showing frequent smudge marks. Two volumes. Size is 8.27 inch (21 cm) h. × 5.12 inch (13 cm) w.

1889(?) Edition. The date of publication is not given on this site, but the title using the words "Illustrated" (*tukao* 圖考) appeared on editions issued in 1886 and 1889. In *Medical Therapies Illustrated* (*Fanzheng tukao* 翻症圖考), Shenyutang *zi* 慎餘堂梓. Seventy-four therapies are listed in this work. The copy was located in Shandong province, Dezhou city 山東省德州市. Size is 7.01 inch (18 cm) h. × 4.33 inch (11 cm) w. Appears to have 38 folio pages. See http://book.kongfz.com/357294/3052552727/, accessed July 28, 2021. No longer available as of November 2023.

Another title put out by this publishing house was the *Yijing* 易經 of the Zhou Dynasty (*Zhou Yi* 周易) with publication information listed on its title page as "Shenyutang textbook" (*Shenyutang keben* 慎餘堂課本). This was a woodblock edition with text of large and clear characters, with intertext commentary and top-of-page notes, though some pages showed much ink smudging. The site listed this title size as 9.4 inch (24 cm) h. × 5.9 inch (15 cm) w. However, in its explanation of provenance, the site said this was issued by Shenyitang 慎怡堂, a Qing-era publisher located in Jiangxi province, Qingjiang-xian 江西省清江縣. Found on https://www.ruten.com.tw/item/show?22025719516561, accessed December 28, 2021, and November 29, 2023.

1891 Edition. *Elaborations on Medical Therapies* (*Xiuxiang fanzheng* 繡像翻症). Published as a woodblock edition by Yishantang 義善堂, *Guangxu shiqi nian* 光緒十七年 (1891). The edition is described as having an *Appendix of Seventy-Four Different Therapies Illustrated* (*Futu miaohui qishisi zhong butong xingtai fanzheng* 附圖描繪七十四不同形態翻症), but it is unclear if this was part of the printed title or was simply a continuation of the printed pages. Listed in *Chinese Dictionary of Medical Books* (*Zhongguo yiji da cidian* 中國醫籍大辭典), ed. the Compilation Committee (*Bianzuan weiyuanhui* 編纂委員會), Shanghai Scientific Press (Shanghai kexue jishu chubanshe 上海科學技術出版社), 2002.

1892 Edition. *New Expanded Elaborations on the Seventy-Four Medical Therapies; Appendix of Forty Miraculous Old Therapies* (*Xinzeng xiuxiang qishisi fanzheng; houfu miaofang sishi yizhong* 新增繡像七十四翻症；後附妙方四十遺

種). Published as a woodblock edition by Damingtang *zi* 大明堂梓, *Guangxu shiba nian* 光緒十八年 (1892). The appendix is titled *Elaborations on Therapies* (*Xiuxiang fanzheng* 繡像翻症), earlier published by the Wenhuatang *zi* 文華堂梓 in *Tongzhi qi nian* 同治七年 (1868). The online version is a woodblock edition. Many pages are fully illustrated in this posting. The size was listed as 7.87 inch (20 cm) h. × 5.51 inch (14 cm) w. See http://book.kongfz. com/27537/2872464036/, accessed July 2021. This site was closed as of January 3, 2022. Site no longer active as of December 2023.

1903 Edition. *Elaborations on Medical Therapies* (*Xiuxiang fanzheng* 繡像翻症). Woodblock held by Shudetang *zi* 樹德堂梓. Newly cut in 1903 (*Guangxu guimao xinke* 光緒癸卯新刻). This has thirty-nine folio pages. A woodblock edition with many ink smudge marks. Accessed August 2021. Available in Taiwan at the National Palace Museum (*Guoli gugong bowuyuan* 國立故宮博物院). This version, in its illustrations and sequence of therapies, is similar to my copy of the manual which is translated in this book. The drawings, however, were done by a different artist. I thank the National Palace Museum for their assistance to me in viewing this copy online.

The links below lead you into the National Palace Museum website, and from there one can search out specific titles of the collection: http://rbk-doc. npm.edu.tw/npmtpc/npmtpall?@@0.19882639106647204 (click on *shanben guji* 善本古籍); https://www.npm.gov.tw/Sitemap.aspx?sno=01000008&l=2; 國立故宮博物院圖書文獻數位典藏資料庫: http://rbk-doc.npm.edu.tw/npmtpc/npmtpall.

Uncertain Year Edition. *Capital Edition Seventy-Two Therapies* (*Jingdu qishier fan* 京都七十二翻). This is how the title is listed on the website. This woodblock edition was printed on very thin paper so the pages have been reinforced by slipping a paper between the folded folio pages. The printed type on the inserted paper is in the simplified form (*jiantizi* 簡體字), and appears to be contemporary or post-1970. The title pages with publication information are missing, but hand-written on the back cover with a marking pen are the words "Seventy-Two Medical Therapies for a Body in Pain" (*Tongzheng shen 72 fanzheng* 痛症身72翻症). The site listing clarifies that only sixty medical recipes remain in this edition. The original pages appear to be from an earlier, probably a Qing-era printing. The size of 7.24 inch (18.4 cm) h. × 5.12 inch (13 cm) w. This copy was located in Shandong province, Heze city 山東省菏

澤市. See https://book.kongfz.com/38542/1117282838/, accessed July 2021. This site was closed as of January 3, 2022, and accessible on April 17, 2024.

Hand-Written Copies

China had a vibrant manuscript culture that continued well into the 1950s. In early China, manuscripts were circulated in hand-written form, so a person wishing to own a book would often copy out the entire manuscript by hand. This was considered a good way to read the book and to thoroughly learn its contents well. It was also possible to employ a scholar, student, or scribe to copy the manuscript. By the late 1800s many books had been printed using either woodblocks or the more recently imported lithography method. Most of those books were illustrated, were available throughout the country (though with uncertain distribution), and were relatively inexpensive.

Nevertheless, in spite of the proliferation of printed books, many people continued to copy out texts by hand. The *Seventy-Two Therapies* (*Qishier fanzheng* 七十二翻症) was one of those titles. When a book was copied by hand, very often there was no date or place of publication recorded. In trying to determine a likely date for when the copy was made, we look first at the paper used to try to determine the age of the copy. We also look at the binding, usually string or twine, to try to determine the quality of the resources put into making the copy. Poor quality paper with noticeable impurities or badly browned indicates the copier was a person of lower economic status and was using materials of inferior quality. String was considered more valuable for binding because it could also be used to mend clothes. We can examine the quality of the drawings, writing, and skill at using the brush to get an idea of the educational level of the person doing the copy work.

The hand-written copies I located for sale on the internet seem to have been produced from the 1920s down to the late 1950s. These were available in 2021 when I was doing this research. The two copies I located both used the title "Elaborations on Medical Therapies" (*Xiuxiang fanzheng* 繡像翻症), which was the title used on many of the most widely circulated copies of this title from the late Qing through the Republican period.

Hand-Written Copy (*Shouxieben* 手寫本). "Seventy-Two Therapies" (*Qishier fanzheng* 七十二翻症). The seller Kongfuzi Bookstore gives the date of this

manuscript as 1820. It is 24 folio pages in a size of 8.6 inch (22 cm) h. ×
6.10 inch (15.5 cm) w. This is all text with no illustrations, and no date is
written on the manuscript. It was located in Shandong province, Dezhou
city 山東省德州市. It is not possible to confirm an 1820 date for this copy
based on the online photos of the pages shown. See https://book.kongfz.
com/357294/4488478200/, accessed December 4, 2023.

Hand-Written Copy (*Shouxieben* 手寫本). "Elaborations on Medical Therapies" (*Xiuxiang fanzheng* 繡像翻症). This is a hand-written copy of 16 folio
pages that contain prescriptions along with the simply-drawn person in distress and a corresponding animal. In writing out the title, the person who
copied this wrote Capital Taishan Bookstore (*Jingdu Taishantang* 京都泰山
堂). This copy was located in Henan province, Anyang city 河南省安陽市.
Also written on the first page: "Elaborations on Medical Therapies" (*Xiuxiang*
繡像), "Seventy-Two Therapies" (*Qishier fanzheng* 七十二翻症); "Illustrations
of Therapies" (*Fanzheng tukao* 翻症圖考), "Seventy-Two Types of Remedies"
(*Qishier zhong zhifa* 七十二種治法), and "Paralysis" (*Tanjing* 癱經). Note some
characters using the simplified style. Simplified styles of writing were often
used by members of the public prior to 1950 when writing letters or keeping notebooks. The simplifications formed the basis of the more systematic
and expanded simplification of characters carried out by the Chinese government in the 1950s. This copy appears to be on machine-made paper,
which could mean a date of 1930s to 1950s. This may have been written with
a ball-point pen, giving a date of 1940s or later. See http://book.kongfz.
com/181274/3302720698/, accessed July 2021. Appears to be no longer available in November 2023.

Hand-Written Copy (*Shouxieben* 手寫本). Listed as "Elaborations of Therapies" (*Xiuxiang fanzheng* 繡像翻症). Hand-written on the cover: "Seventy-Four
Therapies" (*Fanzheng qishisi tiao* 翻症柒拾肆條). Simple but clear wording and
illustrations are in this copy. The complete form of characters are used. The
pages are illustrated on the posting; thirty-six therapies are given. Possibly
written on machine-made paper, which could give a date of post-1900 on, with
one page having ink blots similar to leaky ink pens from the 1930s through to
the 1950s in China. On a photo of the cover, a partial date (the second character can only be inferred) that appears to be *guichou* 癸丑 can be seen (see

Appendix B). The most likely date would then be 1973. The next likely *gui-chou* year would be 1913. Approximate size: 7.87 inch (20 cm) h. × 5.51 inch (14 cm) w. See https://book.kongfz.com/135932/2500258193/, accessed July 2021. Still open in December 2023.

Lithographed Editions of the Republican Period

In 1916 there was a popular renewed interest in China about this collection of medical recipes. Chinese publishers, principally in Beijing and Shanghai, began issuing lithographed copies of the collection. Some of the publishers had new illustrations made. This means that in some illustrations the drawings show patients wearing clothing and with a hairstyle that would have been common in the Qing era. In the 1916 lithographs, however, some of the newer illustrations show men (usually the figures are men, although a few females appear) with Western-style hairstyles and clothing likely to have been worn in China in the early 1900s. Many of the versions of this collection available today in mainland China, Taiwan, and held by libraries outside of China are reprints of these 1916 editions. The editions I located are listed separately below.

1916 Edition. *Illustrated Acupuncture Made Easy; Appendix of Seventy-Two Therapies Illustrated and Explained (Huitu yixue; fu qishier fan tushuo* 繪圖易學；附七十二番圖説*)* from Guangyi Publishing House (*Guangyi shuju* 廣益書局) held by University of Hong Kong. I thank the University of Hong Kong Library for providing me with a xeroxed copy of this title. One of the first publishing companies in China to bring out this new lithographed edition was *Guangyi shuju*. The company was formed in 1900 in Shanghai by Wei Tiansheng 魏天生, Du Mingyan 杜鳴雁, and Xiao Bairun 蕭佰潤. Among its co-founders was Li Dongsheng 李東生. It was sometimes called the Guangyi Book Studio (*Guangyi shushi* 廣益書室), but adopted the *Guangyi shuju* name by 1903. Its marketing plan was to publish books classified as *keju kaochang* 科舉考場, which meant academic texts of Chinese traditional subjects used to prepare for the imperial examinations, which had been discontinued in 1905 but were still considered important classical texts by many people. They would also publish books pertaining to elementary education for children (*tongmeng duwu* 童蒙讀物). Until 1937 it published many popular titles of novels, stories, and reprinted older

illustrated classics on medicine, fortunetelling, and Chinese classical literature. By the late 1930s its books were put out in cheap and often discounted
paperback editions, often with multiple typos. The Japanese occupation of
Shanghai from 1937 brought its business to a close.

The company managed to reorganize itself in 1943 with an influx of
capital. The chairman of its board was Wei Bingrong 魏炳榮 and its executive
director was Liu Jikang 劉季康. Its staff of 37 began issuing popular novels.
In 1947 it joined with four other publishers to begin issuing school textbooks.
The combined editorial and printing resources of the group of five allowed
them to open at least ten branches throughout China. Their books were
put out in lithographed and typeset editions. After 1950 the company was
absorbed into other publishing units.

The title of the Guangyi Publishing House 1916 reprint listed here was
a lithograph copy of a 1798 woodblock printed edition titled *Illustrated Acupuncture Made Easy* (*Huitu zhenjiu yixue* 繪圖針灸易學) by Li Shouxian 李守先
(1735–1809), first printed in the third year of the *Jiaqing* 嘉慶 reign period of
the Qing Dynasty (*Daqing Jiaching san nian* 大清嘉慶三年, 1798). The second
title (referred to as a *juan* 卷) was *Seventy-Two Therapies Completely Illustrated*
(*Qishier fan quantu* 七十二翻全圖). It had been compiled by Li Shouxian's students and had been added to this collection as an appendix in *Guangxu ershiqi
nian* 光緒二十七年 (1847) with the title of *Seventy-Two Therapies Illustrated*
(*Qishier fan tu* 七十二翻圖). Subsequently both titles in lithographed form were
regularly published together and continue today to be issued together usually
under the title of *Illustrated Acupuncture Made Easy* (*Huitu zhenjiu yixue* 繪圖針
灸易學).

A copy of the Guangyi Publishing House 1916 edition is, as stated above,
held by University of Hong Kong Library. In this copy of the book, the publishers added folio page 2 in its proper location (following folio page 1), but then
reprinted the same page at the end of the publication, following folio page 12.
This "inattention" perhaps indicates the somewhat sloppy production work
associated with issuing "pirated" editions. The illustrations in this edition all
show figures with a post-Qing hairstyle. Further, none of the figures shows
Qing-era outer clothing, so these illustrations were done in the Republican
period after the fall of the Qing Dynasty.

A link for a copy of this title is on the Kongfuzi Bookstore is https://book.
kongfz.com/172359/2921307533/, accessed December 18, 2021. Still open in
December 2023.

1916 Wellcome Edition. *Illustrated Acupuncture Made Easy (Huitu zhenjiu yixue* 繪圖針灸易學*).* A lithographed edition of the *Seventy-Two Therapies* titled *Seventy-Two Therapies All Illustrated (Qishier fan quantu* 七十二翻全圖*)* was acquired and put online by the Wellcome Collection Museum and Library, London. They seem to show a lithographed version of a woodblock edition. The illustrations all show Qing-era hairstyles and Qing-era outer clothing. These lithographed drawings were taken from earlier Qing editions. The publication information and date are not available on the site, although a librarian at Wellcome told me it was a 1916 publication. No size is given. See https://wellcomecollection.org/works/xhxbarf4, accessed July 2021, and December 12, 2023.

1916 Edition. *Illustrated Acupuncture Made Easy; Appendix of Illustrated Seventy-Two Therapies (Huitu zhenjiu yixue; fu qishier fan quantu* 繪圖針灸易學；附七十二翻全圖*),* Shanghai Guangyi Publishing House *(Shanghai Guangyi shuju* 上海廣益書局*), Minguo wu nian* 民國五年 (1916). See https://wantubizhi.com/image.aspx?w=, accessed August 2021. No longer available as of November 2023.

1916 Edition. *Illustrated Acupuncture Made Easy (Huitu zhenjiu yixue* 繪圖針灸易學*),* with the title *Seventy-Two Therapies Completely Illustrated (Qishier fan quantu* 七十二翻全圖*)* published as an appendix *(fu* 附*).* The book ends following the appendix. Lithographed reprint issued by Shanghai Guangyi Publishing House *(Shanghai Guangyi shuju* 上海廣益書局*).* Its size is listed 7.99 inch (20.3 cm) h. × 5.19 inch (13.2 cm) w. Many of the pages are illustrated. In summer 2021 this was available at the Kongfuzi Bookstore for RMB 1,300. http://book.kongfz.com/3240/852511409/. Site still open in December 2023. The illustrations in this edition are different from those in the Guangyi Publishing House edition held in the Wellcome Collection. A lithographed 1916 Guangyi edition showing the afflicted wearing Western-style haircuts is at https://book.kongfz.com/12820/6430725597/, accessed December 2023.

1916 Edition. This edition was reprinted in Taiwan in 1997. It was a reprint of *Illustrated Acupuncture Made Easy (Huitu zhenjiu yixue* 繪圖針灸易學*),* with the title *Seventy-Two Therapies Completely Illustrated (Qishier fan quantu* 七十二翻全圖*)* published as an appendix *(fu* 附*).* Published in Taipei by Xinwenfeng Printing Company *(Xinwenfeng chuban gongsi* 新文豐出版公司*)* and listed below under the 1997 Taiwan re-issue. The original publisher and date of publication are not given on the reprinted version.

1916 Edition. *Illustrated Acupuncture Made Easy, Two Volumes; Appendix of Seventy-Two Therapies Completely Illustrated* (*Huitu zhenjiu yixue, shangxia juan; fu qishier fan quantu* 繪圖針灸易學，上下卷；附七十二翻全圖), three volumes, by Li Shouxian 李守先 (1735–1809). Published in Shanghai by the Cuiying Book Company (*Cuiying shuju* 萃英書局).

The Shanghai Cuiying Book Company was founded in the *Guangxu* 光緒 era (1875–1908) of the Qing Dynasty. The company was very active from 1912 to 1926. Among the titles they concentrated on were medical-related topics and textbooks. They also issued lithographed editions of a number of earlier Qing period woodblock publications. This appears to be the copy held by the Rare Books Collection of the Harvard-Yenching Library at Harvard, which does not have the date of publication. The publication has 12 folio pages. Its price was listed as "Each copy 30 cents big money" (*meibu dingjia dayang sanjiao* 每部定價大洋叁角). The phrase *dayang* 大洋 ("large foreign") was used at the end of the Qing Dynasty and in the Republican period (roughly between the 1880s and the 1940s) by the common people to refer to Western types of coins or bills that had been introduced to China by the Western powers to replace Chinese traditional currencies. I was able to examine this copy at the Harvard-Yenching Library Rare Books Room in 2021.

1918 Edition. *Illustrated Acupuncture Made Easy; Appendix of Seventy-Two Therapies Illustrated and Explained* (*Huitu zhenjiu yixue; fu qishierfan tushuo* 繪圖針灸易學；附七十二翻圖説), Zhuji Book Company (*Zhuji shuju* 鑄記書局), *Minguo qi nian* 民國七年 (1918). Found on https://wantubizhi.com by searching "舊書," "七十二翻症," or "民間七十二翻症圖解," accessed July 2021. Through this link I found a photo of two pages of the 1918 edition, listed on 7788.com, accessed December 18, 2021. Wantubizhi.com (*wantubizhi wang* 萬圖壁紙網) advertises and sells items from other merchants.

The Zhuji Book Company has a long history as a publisher of reference books and academic titles. Its predecessor was the Hubei Lexicographic (Dictionary) Publishing Company (*Hubei cishu chubanshe* 湖北辭書出版社) set up in 1885. It began publishing as an independent entity in 1892 and changed its name to Foundry of Records Publishing Company (*Zhuji shuju* 鑄記書局)

in 1902. It continues operations today, with its staff of 43 producing such current titles as *Chinese Character Dictionary* (*Hanyu dazidian* 漢語大字典), *Complete Dictionary of Chinese Idioms* (*Zhonghua chengyu quandian* 中華成語全典), *Complete Dictionary of Tang Dynasty Poetic Allusions* (*Quan Tangshi diangu cidian* 全唐詩典故辭典), and nearly 100 other titles annually. It is interesting to note that this serious and respected publisher decided to issue its own edition of *Acupuncture Made Easy* (*Zhenjiu yixue* 針灸易學) with its appendix of the *Seventy-Two Therapies*, indicating that this title was still selling well and was popular with the educated public. This was done following the 1916 issue of the same title by at least two other Chinese publishers, *Guangyi shuju* 廣益書局 and *Cuiying shuju* 萃英書局. In the 1918 edition, the publisher had new illustrations made of afflicted patients. None of these had the traditional Qing hairstyle. See https://wantubizhi.com/image350909353514.html, accessed December 28, 2021. Unavailable as of December 2023.

1939 Edition. *Illustrated Acupuncture Made Easy, Two Volumes; Appendix of Seventy-Two Therapies Completely Illustrated* (*Huitu zhenjiu yixue, shangxia juan; fu qishier fan quantu* 繪圖針灸易學，上下卷；附七十二翻全圖). Published in Baoding 保定: Xiaozhong Book Company (*Xiaozhong shuju* 曉鐘書局), *Zhonghua minguo ershiba nian* 中華民國二十八年 (1939). This appears to be a reprint of an 1886 edition put out in *Guangxu shier nian* 光緒十二年. 10.35 inch (26.3 cm) h. × 5.43 inch (13.8 cm) w. See https://www.qudiandi.com/product/item/pid/10083849.html, accessed July 2021; https://www.qudiandi.com/product/item/pid/10061934.htm, accessed August 2021 and December 2023.

Lithographed editions of *Acupuncture Made Easy*, probably containing the *Seventy-Two Therapies*, were issued several times in the early People's Republic. Those were in 1951 by the Chinese Medicine Bookstore (*Zhongyi shuju* 中醫書局); in 1951 by the Constructing Literature Bookstore (*Jianwen shuju* 建文書局); and in 1954 by the Shanghai Jinzhang Bookstore (*Shanghai Jinzhang shuju* 上海錦章書局), then reproduced by the Beijing China Bookstore (*Beijing Zhongguo shudian* 北京中國書店). I have not seen copies of any of these editions. These editions are listed in Xu Jingsheng, ed., *Acupuncture Made Easy: Annotated* (*Zhenjiu yixue: Jiaozhu* 針灸易學：校注). The editors of this book appear to have used editions from the *Guangyi shuju* 廣益書局 (1916), *Jianwen shuju* 建文書局 (1951), and *Jinzhang shuju* 錦章書局 (1954), as references for the proofread text that appears in their book. The 1950s reprint editions are mentioned in Gao Xiyan 高希言 et al., annot., Xu Jingsheng 許敬生, ed., *Acupuncture Made Easy: Annotated* (*Zhenjiu yixue: Jiaozhu* 針灸易學：校注), Zhengzhou: Henan kexue jishu chubanshe 河南科學技術出版社, 2017, p. 6.

Text-Only Version. *Chinese Folk Medicine The Seventy-Two Therapies, by the Simple Medicine and Massage Group* (*Minjian Zhongyi qishier fan; zuozhe: Yiyi tuinapai* 民間中醫七十二翻；作者：易醫推拿派). This Chinese text version was put online by Nanchizi 南池子. Original publication information on this published edition is not given. See http://blog.sina.com.cn/s/blog_513a59070102vds1.html, accessed July 2021. It was posted on April 1, 2015, and possibly can be found in the listing of the posts on the site: "民間中醫七十二翻_風一樣的男孩_新浪博客." The site concerns itself with all sorts of health and health-related issues, among which this title became one for a time. This title in a lithographed, possibly 1916 edition, can still be found on the site through searching and some pages are available to be seen. Accessed December 2023.

Printed Editions in Taiwan and the Mainland China

A number of libraries in the United States and around the world hold copies of these reprinted versions. I have not tracked down all of these reprints. I am inclined to say that they are of one of the 1916 lithographed versions listed above. Most likely they are reprints of the same lithographic plates used by each Taiwan publisher in turn.

1969 Edition. *Illustrated Acupuncture Made Easy* (*Huitu zhenjiu yixue* 繪圖針灸易學). Note that these reprinted editions include the *Seventy-Two Therapies* (*Qishier fanzheng* 七十二翻症). Published in Taipei by Basic Education Book Company (*Qiye shuju* 啟業書局).

The Qiye Book Company was set up in 1965 in Taipei. I assume Taiwan had the plates of an earlier mainland print run or used a copy of this title they had on hand to republish this book. In the late 1950s and 1960s publishers in Taiwan reprinted many titles previously issued in the 1930s and 1940s on the mainland. Book copyright laws were not in effect in Taiwan at that time. When those Taiwan reprinted books, originally from the 1930s and reprinted in the 1950s or 1960s, became available in the Liulichang 琉璃廠 antiques district in Beijing in the 1980s, they could be quite expensive. The 1969 Taipei edition cited here was seen as an educational textbook for students, thus it was put out by the imprint of the Basic Education Book Company.

1973 Edition. *Illustrated Acupuncture Made Easy* (*Huitu zhenjiu yixue* 繪圖針灸易學). Note that these reprinted editions include the *Seventy-Two Therapies* (*Qishier fanzheng* 七十二翻症). Two 1973 print runs were published in Taipei by Southwest Book Company (*Xinan shuju* 西南書局).

The Xinan Book Company was set up to publish textbooks for junior and high school students. We can assume the Xinan Book Company decided to do a marketing campaign with this title to get sales from it. They were successful and the book had a second print run in 1973.

1978 Edition. *Illustrated Acupuncture Made Easy* (*Huitu zhenjiu yixue* 繪圖針灸易學). Note that these reprinted editions include the *Seventy-Two Therapies* (*Qishier fanzheng* 七十二翻症). Published in Taipei by Lixing Book Company (*Lixing shuju* 力行書局).

The Lixing Company was set up in 1951 when it published dictionaries, medical titles, and textbooks. But in the past thirty years since the 1990s it has expanded to be an office supply company, with stationery, laptops, and supplies used by professional artists.

Five years after the reprint edition of *Acupuncture Made Easy* put out by the Xinan Book Company in Taipei, the Lixing Book Company in Taipei reissued it under their imprint, to take their turn in getting sales from the title.

1979 Edition. *Illustrated Acupuncture Made Easy* (*Huitu zhenjiu yixue* 繪圖針灸易學). Note that these reprinted editions include the *Seventy-Two Therapies* (*Qishier fanzheng* 七十二翻症). Reprinted in Taipei by the Xinan Book Company.

Xinan Book Company realized that the Lixing Book Company had experienced good sales with their 1978 edition of the title, so Xinan once again issued their earlier 1973 edition.

1985 Edition. *Illustrated Acupuncture Made Easy* (*Huitu zhenjiu yixue* 繪圖針灸易學). Note that these reprinted editions include the *Seventy-Two Therapies* (*Qishier fanzheng* 七十二翻症). Published in Beijing by Beijing China Bookstore (*Beijing Zhongguo shudian* 北京中國書店).

In 1985 China was awaking from its thirty-five years, since 1950, of politically and ideologically imposed restraints on all aspects of daily life. This awakening meant a less fettered reappreciation of China's history and culture.

Although the Beijing China Bookstore is a nation-wide chain, still these days (I write this in 2022) often titles published by one of its branches are not easily available nor are they displayed in other branches of the chain. I was told this at the Beijing branch of one of these chain bookstores in 2013, after asking about a title I was interested in. Thus, this reprinted title was probably not widely available in China at the time. An electronic version was also available from the publisher. A printed copy for sale is listed on https://book.kongfz.com/213727/6565211826/, accessed December 2023. Another copy can be found at https://book.kongfz.com/13983/6522691977/, accessed December 2023. At https://book.kongfz.com/413068/6454558299/ is a copy located in Chongqing city, Dadukou district 重慶市大渡口區, accessed December 2023. A 1985 edition from Heilongjiang province, Harbin city 黑龍江省哈爾濱市 is at https://book.kongfz.com/191568/5766166485/, accessed December 2023. An inside page from the *Huitu zhenjiu yixue* first section *shangzhuan*, and in the second *qishier fanzheng* section, shows the afflicted males dressing their hair in the Qing style.

1991 Edition. *Illustrated Acupuncture Made Easy* (*Huitu zhenjiu yixue* 繪圖針灸易學*). Note that these reprinted editions include the *Seventy-Two Therapies* (*Qishier fanzheng* 七十二翻症). Republished in Beijing by Beijing China Bookstore (*Beijing Zhongguo shudian* 北京中國書店).

By 1991, the People's Republic was undergoing an ever-strengthening reappraisal of its past and its thinking about its future social, economic, and cultural trajectory. The reissue of this title was a good symbol of those trends showing a willingness for the public to think about earlier times. The 1991 version using simplified characters is at https://book.kongfz.com/19219/6547227788/, accessed December 2023. A copy located in Beijing, Changping district 北京市昌平區 is at https://book.kongfz.com/23112/6453340258/, accessed December 2023. A copy of this edition from Beijing, Shijingshan district 北京市石景山區 is at https://book.kongfz.com/233421/6178102235/, accessed December 2023. A 1991 edition from Henan province, Xinyang city 河南省信陽市 is at https://book.kongfz.com/24101/6352853389/, accessed December 2023.

1997 Edition. *Illustrated Acupuncture Made Easy* (*Huitu zhenjiu yixue* 繪圖針灸易學). Note that these reprinted editions include the *Seventy-Two Therapies*

Completely Illustrated (*Qishier fanzheng quantu* 七十二翻症全圖). Published in Taipei by Xinwenfeng Printing Company (*Xinwenfeng chuban gongsi* 新文豐出版公司).

Xinwenfeng was established in 1973 to publish titles and collections of materials on many aspects of Chinese culture including Confucianism, Buddhism, Daoism, folk culture, etc. It is proud of its more than fifty-year history.

The 1997 version of *Illustrated Acupuncture Made Easy* is listed in this bibliography above as originally a 1916 edition. The Xinwenfeng edition contains a reprint of the original 1798 preface by Li Shouxian for the *Illustrated Acupuncture Made Easy* (*Huitu zhenjiu yixue* 繪圖針灸易學) and it also contains a reprint of a preface from 1847, the year the *Seventy-Two Medical Therapies Completely Illustrated* (*Qishier fan quantu* 七十二翻全圖) was compiled. The *Seventy-Two Therapies* are illustrated on pages 69–78 of the reprinted version. This preface was written by Xu Tianxi 許天錫. In the illustrations for the medical therapies some of the male figures no longer wear the required Qing style of hairdo, so these illustrations were drawn after the end of the Qing. This reprint contains seventy-six therapies. The medical recipes have basic punctuation, same as was used in other 1916 editions of the title. It is possible that all of the Taiwan reprints since the 1969 edition are of the same woodblocks or lithographic plates, but I have not been able to see all of the Taiwan or PRC reprinted editions.

This Xinwenfeng reprinting has removed the information about the publisher who originally issued his volume in 1916. However, this appears to be a reprint of the 1916 edition of these titles issued by *Shanghai Guangyi shuju* 上海廣益書局. The *Seventy-Two Therapies* are titled *Qishier fan tu* 七十二翻圖, and in the reprint they follow folio page 27 of Volume 2 (*juanxia* 卷下) of the title work. The *Seventy-Two Therapies* are on folio pages 2 to 5 of this second *juan*. They are followed in the Xinwenfeng reprint by the title *Acupuncture Questions and Answers* (*Zhenjiu wenda* 針灸問答) by Wang Ji 汪機. Wang Ji (1463–1539) was a Ming physician who published on medical issues. His life and contributions are studied in the book by Joanna Grant, *A Chinese Physician: Wang Ji and the Stone Mountain Medical Case Histories* (London: Routledge, 2003).

The original woodblock edition is listed as having a size of 7.9 inch (20.3 cm) h. × 5.2 inch (13.2 cm) w. The Xinwenfeng reprint is about the same size as the original.

The *Xinwenfeng* classification considers this to be a textbook for elementary and junior high school students, similar to the classification given to the initial Taiwan printing by *Qiye shuju* 啟業書局 in 1969. Does this mean it is considered not for use by pharmacists or the adult population?

2016 Edition. *Illustrated Acupuncture Made Easy* (*Huitu zhenjiu yixue* 繪圖針灸易學). Note that these reprinted editions include the *Seventy-Two Therapies* (*Qishier fanzheng* 七十二翻症). *Illustrated Acupuncture Made Easy*, 3 Volumes (*Huitu zhenjiu yixue, san juan* 繪圖針灸易學，三卷) by Li Shouxian 李守先. Published in Beijing by Beijing Erudition Digital Technology Research Center (*Beijing Airusheng shuzihuajishu yanjiu zhongxin* 北京愛如生數字化技術研究中心), 2016. Electronic (digitalized) version.

The Beijing Erudition Digital Technology Research Center was set up in 1998 as the Beijing Erudition Cultural Exchange Company, Ltd. (*Beijing Airusheng wenhua jiaoliu youxiangongsi* 北京愛如生文化交流有限公司), and changed to its present name in 2003. Its purpose was to digitalize traditional Chinese books, and to that end it developed its own digitalization software. It relied on Peking University, Tsinghua University, and the Chinese Academy of Sciences for grants to allow the digitalization project to begin. Since then it has created at least fourteen large-scale databases and has digitalized hundreds of titles, including one million pieces from the Ming and Qing archives, and 3,000 titles of modern newspapers and periodicals. These Erudition digital products have been sold to twenty-four domestic provinces, municipalities, and autonomous regions within mainland China and to eleven countries. The products have been purchased by national libraries and major universities in Taiwan, Japan, South Korea, New Zealand, Germany, Britain, France, the United States, and Canada. This includes the Library of Congress in the United States, the National Library of Berlin, the Toyo Bunko in Japan, Peking University, University of Hong Kong, Harvard University, Oxford University, Waseda University in Japan, etc.

It was bound to come to this. A fully electronic version. No paper needed. Nevertheless, the enduring importance of this collection of insights on medical problems and observations initially compiled in the late 1700s was demonstrated by having this title included in the digitalization project.

IMAGES AND
THE *SEVENTY-TWO THERAPIES*

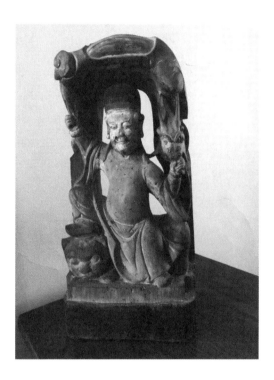

The most prominent of the early physicians and the one best known to the Chinese people today is Sun Simiao 孫思邈. He lived during the Sui and Tang Dynasties (581–907 CE) and is said to have died in 682 CE. Many legends have grown up around him. He once extracted a bone that had been caught in a tiger's throat and in gratitude the tiger became his protector, as seen in this wooden carved figure. At another time he rescued the son of the Dragon King from a beating given by a shepherd. We see him here with a dragon in close proximity. It is possible the figure's right hand once held a needle, symbolic of the use of acupuncture. Sun Simiao is venerated as the King of Medicine (*Yaowang* 藥王). This figure is in my personal collection. Author photo.

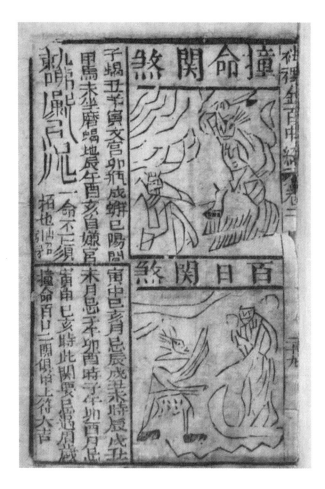

This is an illustration that helped me determine the probable date of the manual translated in this book. This photo is a page of a woodblock edition of *Pocket Edition of Precious Accurate Information; Imperial Calendar Almanac* (*Xiuli Jinbaizhongjing; Yuding wannianli* 袖裏金百中經；御定萬年曆). The calendar section in this almanac covers the years 1848 to 1864, which tells me it was printed in 1848 and was very likely still circulating in the 1860s. I surmise the artist who made those drawings in the mid-1800s was the same person who illustrated my edition of the *Seventy-Two Therapies*. Notice the somewhat abstract and impressionistic use of lines. The figures on this page are the troublesome goblins (*sha* 煞) that impede one's passage through the difficulties, called gates or passes (*guan* 關), which human beings may encounter during the course of their lives. The almanac is in my personal collection. Author photo.

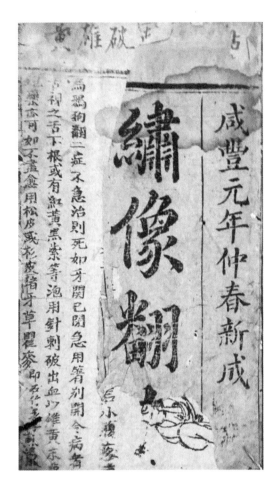

Front page of the 1851 edition of the *Elaborations on Medical Therapies* (*Xiuxiang fanzheng* 繡像翻症) published by Wenlintang 文林堂 issued in *Xianfeng yuannian er yue* 咸豐元年二月 (February 1851). Next to the title in large characters is the date of publication: "Newly Published Late Spring 1851" (*Xianfeng yuannian zhongchun xincheng* 咸豐元年仲春新成). On the page facing the title page are notations of a doctor who was consulting the *Seventy-Two Therapies*. He appears to have been writing an herbal recipe containing medically useful herbs such as angelica (*danggui* 當歸), ginseng (*renshen* 人參), and the Notopterygium Root (*qianghuo* 羌活). These were possibly to use for a decoction called Angelica and Notopterygium (*Danggui qianghuo tang* 當歸羌活湯) that could be used for stroke patients with heat (*re* 熱) symptoms such as cough and excessive phlegm. Image by Kongfz.com.

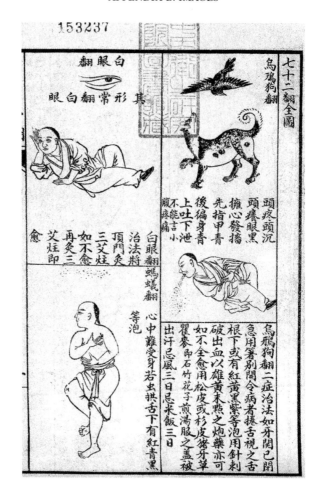

This is a page from the 1916 lithographed edition of the *Seventy-Two Therapies* from the book titled *Illustrated Acupuncture Made Easy* (*Huitu zhenjiu yixue* 繪圖針灸易學) put online by the Wellcome Collection Museum and Library, London. It shows a lithographed version of a woodblock edition. The Wellcome site lists this work as *Early C20 Chinese Lithograph: "Fan" Diseases.* The illustrations all show Qing-era hairstyles and Qing-era outer clothing. These drawings were taken from earlier Qing editions. No punctuation is visible. The Wellcome site did not show the printed title or publication information. The first title on top right corner of the page reads *Seventy-Two Therapies All Illustrated* (*Qishier fan quantu* 七十二翻全圖). The first column, reading from the right, illustrates the Crow and Dog Therapy (*Wuya gou fan* 烏鴉狗翻). At the top left column is the White Eye Therapy (*Baiyan fan* 白眼翻). Below that is the Ant Therapy (*Mayi fan* 螞蟻翻). None of these therapies are in the manual translated in this book. Image by Wellcome Collection, https://wellcomecollection.org/works/dq4xwd4m.

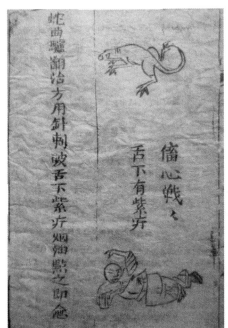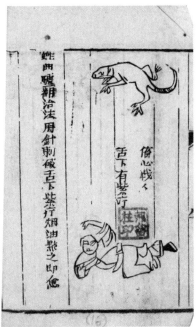

These two pages are a comparison of P16 Donkey Therapy (*Shequlü fan* 蛇曲驢). On our left is the Uncertain Year Edition, listed by the seller as *Capital Edition Seventy-Two Therapies* (*Jingdu qishier fan* 京都七十二翻). It was woodblock printed on very thin paper. On our right is the page from the woodblock printed manual translated in this book, folio page 8b. The seal on this page is from one of the owners of the manual, Hao Liugui 郝留桂. The symptoms and the prescribed treatment are the same, as are the two drawings of the animal associated with this disease at the top of the pages and the depiction of the afflicted patient at the bottom. But two different artists drew the images. Neither recipe has any punctuation. Our left is from Kongfz.com. Our right is an author photo.

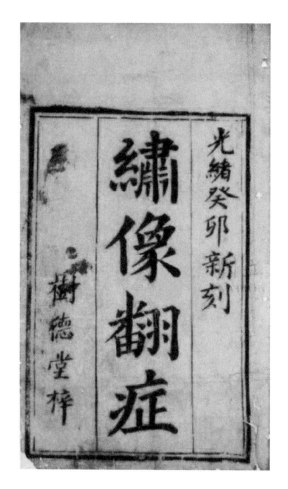

Cover of the 1903 *Elaborations on Medical Therapies* (*Xiuxiang fanzheng* 繡像翻症) published by Shudetang 樹德堂, held by the National Palace Museum (*Guoli gugong bowuyuan* 國立故宮博物院) in Taiwan. This is a woodblock edition showing smudge marks on many pages. The column on our right reads "Newly Cut (Woodblocks) in the *Guimao* Year (1903) of the Guangxu (Emperor)" (*Guangxu guimao xinke* 光緒癸卯新刻). The writing on our left reads "(Woodblocks held / Published) by Shudetang" (*Shudetang zi* 樹德堂梓). Web photo.

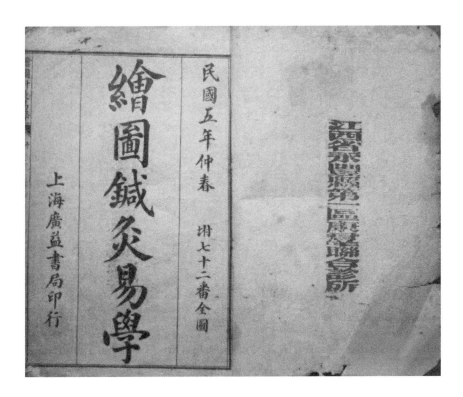

Title page from the *Acupuncture Made Easy; Appendix of the Seventy-Two Therapies Fully Illustrated* (*Huitu zhenjiu yixue; fu qishier fan quantu* 繪圖鍼灸易學；附七十二番全圖), published by the Shanghai Guangyi Publishing House (*Shanghai Guangyi shuju yinxing* 上海廣益書局印行), *Minguo wu nian* 民國五年 (1916).

The red stamp on the facing page reads "Jiangxi Province, Yongfeng County, First District, Public Health United Dispensary" (*Jiangxi-sheng Yongfeng-xian di-yi qu Kangqun lianhe zhensuo* 江西省永豐縣第一區康群聯合診所).

Its size is 7.9 inch (20.3 cm) h. × 5.2 inch (13.2 cm) w. This was the typical size in which the title was usually published. This copy was located in Jiangxi province, Nanchang city (*Jiangxi-sheng Nanchang-shi* 江西省南昌市). The 1997 Taiwan reprint by the Xinwenfeng Printing Company (*Xinwenfeng chuban gongsi* 新文豐出版公司) could have used plates taken from this 1916 edition.

Photo taken from http://book.kongfz.com/3240/852511409/, accessed January 5, 2022, and November 29, 2023.

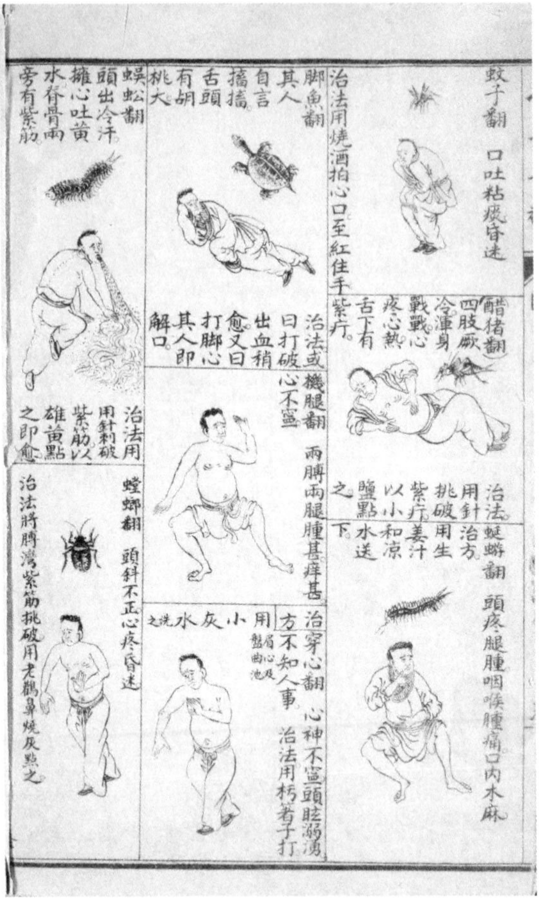

From the 1916 Edition of *Illustrated Acupuncture Made Easy; Appendix of Seventy-Two Therapies Illustrated and Explained* (*Huitu yixue; fu qishier fan tushuo* 繪圖易學；附七十二番圖説) from Guangyitang 廣益堂 held by University of Hong Kong. The figures here all have post-Qing hairstyles. Reading Chinese style starting from the top right corner down the first column, the therapies are: P58 Mosquito Therapy (*Wenzi fan* 蚊子翻), Pickled Pig Therapy (*Cuzhu fan* 醋豬翻), and Slug Therapy (*Yanyou fan* 蜒蝣翻). The middle column reading from the top: Soft-Shelled Turtle Therapy (*Jiaoyu fan* 腳魚翻), Restless Leg Therapy (*Jitui fan* 機腿翻), and P59 Getting to the Heart (Cause) Therapy (*Chuanxin fan* 穿心翻). In the final column on the top left side of the page: P60 Centipede Therapy (*Wugong fan* 蜈蚣翻) and P57 Mantis Therapy (*Tanglang fan* 螳螂翻). Note that not all of the therapies listed here were present in the manual translated in this book. On this illustration we can see a very basic use of punctuation "。" at the end of phrases. Web photo.

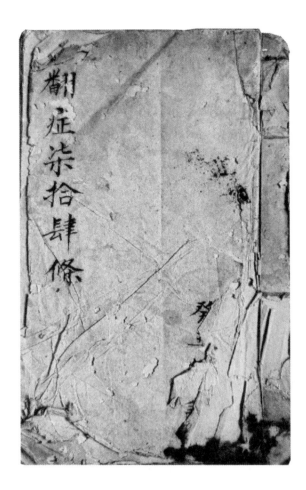

The illustration above shows the cover from a hand-written manuscript listed by the seller as "Elaborations of Therapies" (*Xiuxiang fanzheng* 繡像翻症). Written on the cover: "Seventy-Four Therapies" (*Fanzheng qishisi tiao* 翻症柒拾肆條). On the photo of the cover is a partial date (the second character can only be inferred) that appears to be *guichou* 癸丑. The most likely date would be 1973, though it could also have been 1913. Web photo.

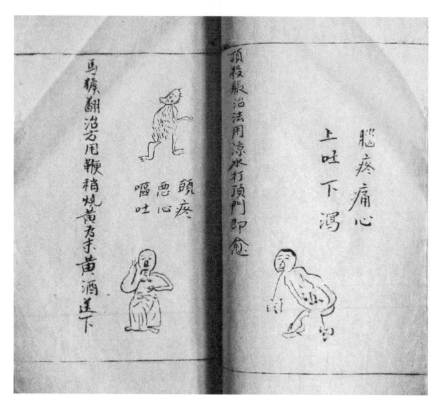

The inside pages written and illustrated by hand from the above book, show on our right P33
"Struggling with Discomfort" (*Dingshazhang fa* 頂殺脹法), and P34 "Horse Monkey Therapy"
(*Mahou fan zhifa* 馬猴翻治法) on our left. Web photo.

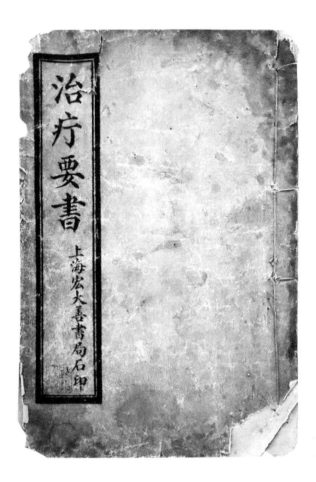

The cover of *Essential for Treating Pustules* (*Zhiding yaoshu* 治疗要書), published by Shanghai Hongda shanshuju 宏大善書局 in 1927. The book was published as a morality book (*shanshu* 善書), which was subscribed by many donations and intended to be given away free to those who would benefit from its contents. This is a lithographed edition taken from an 1870 woodblock version. The book is in my personal collection. Author photo.

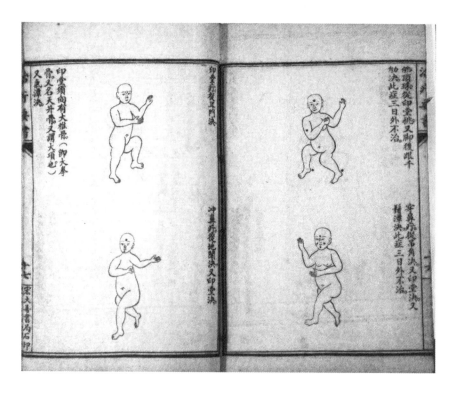

Inside pages from *Essential for Treating Pustules* (*Zhiding yaoshu* 治疗要書), 1927. These pages illustrate the location of certain types of *ding* 疗, which were discolored raised portions on the skin filled with pus or red-purple-black eruptions caused by accumulations of blood. They were similar to pimples, and have been translated as purple boils, blisters, pustules, and sores. Some of the eruptions could be pus-filled and painful. The first (right) page on top shows the *ding* occurring on the forehead where it is called a Jewel on the Buddha's Crown (*fudingzhu* 佛頂珠), and on the bottom Worn on the Nose (*chuanbi* 穿鼻). On page two (left) the top is on the Hall of Impressions (*yintang* 印堂), at the bottom On the Nose (*chongbi* 沖鼻). Author photo.

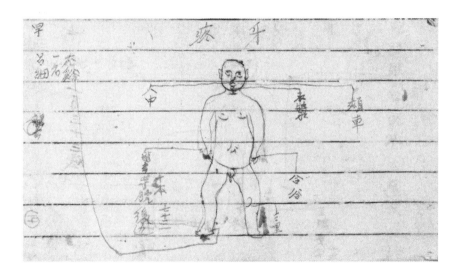

This shows a hand-drawn illustration taken from the hand-written book *Headaches* (*Toutong* 頭痛 / *touteng* 頭疼). This manual in my collection was likely written/drawn by an acupuncturist for his own use. It is filled with line drawings of the human body, each page illustrating the areas where acupuncture needles could be inserted to treat particular conditions. Shown here is the illustration for a toothache (*yateng* 牙疼). It appears from the address given on this book that it was written by a Mr. Liu 劉氏, the owner of the Zhengdetang 政德堂 (a pharmacy or clinic) in Shandong 山東, Jiaozhou-fu 交州府, Taizhuang 台莊, Chengnan 城南. Probably written in the late Qing. Author photo.

BIBLIOGRAPHY

"Acupuncture for Stomach Pain & Bloating." Site of Andrew Hubbard, September 2, 2019. https://drandrewnd.com/acupuncture-for-functional-dyspepsia/. Accessed May 18, 2021.

Acupuncturist's Manual to Relieve Pain: Headache (toutong 頭痛). A manual of 53 pages with illustrations prepared by hand of the proper acupuncture points to use on the body to relieve pains. The practitioner who wrote this left for us his address: Shandong 山東, Yanzhou-fu 兗州府, Ziyang-xian 茲陽縣, Quezi-xiang 卻子鄉, erbao 二保, bajia 八甲, erhu 二戶, which even included his official *baojia* 保甲 designation. He also left the address of the pharmacy he operated, called the Hall of Virtuous Administration (*Zhengdetang* 政德堂). In my personal collection, it was purchased in Qufu 曲阜, Shandong 山東 in April 2009. 7.5 inch (19.05 cm) h. × 5.25 inch (13.34 cm) w. Dated probably early 1900s.

"Ayurvedic Medicine." *Cancer Research UK.* https://www.cancerresearchuk.org/. Accessed April 18, 2022.

Bao Jinjian 寶金劍, ed. *Zhongyi manhua, di-wu ce: Fangji* 中醫漫畫，第五冊：方劑 (*Cartoon TCM, Vol. 5: Medical Prescriptions*). Beijing: Zhongguo kexue jishu chubanshe 中國科學技術出版社, 2018.

Bao Xiangao 鮑相璈. *Raising the Dead and Returning Life: Emergency Medicine of the Qing Dynasty* (*Qisi huisheng* 起死回生). Trans. Lorraine Wilcox. Portland, OR: Chinese Medical Database, 2012.

Bian, He 邊和. *Know Your Remedies: Pharmacy and Culture in Early Modern China.* Princeton, NJ: Princeton University Press, 2020.

Bouhdili, Nadia. "Inside the Mind of an Acupuncturist; How Do We Choose Acupuncture Points?" *Transformational Acupuncture.* July 9, 2015. https://www.dc-acupuncture.com/physical-health/how-acupuncturists-choose-acupuncture-points. Accessed August 2021.

Brokaw, Cynthia J. *Commerce in Culture: The Sibao Book Trade in the Qing and Republican Periods*. Cambridge, MA: Harvard University Asia Center, 2007.

Cao Guowen 曹國文. "Zhongcaoyao zai jindai yangzhuye zhong de yingyong yu yanjiu 中草藥在近代養豬業中的應用與研究" (Research into Chinese Herbal Medicine and the Modern Uses of Raising Pigs). *Sichuan xumu shouyi* 四川畜牧獸醫 (*Szechuan Animal Husbandry and Veterinary Medicine*) 28.11 (2001): 31–32.

Cao Xueqin 曹雪芹. *Dream of the Red Chamber (Cheng Yi Edition)* (*Hongloumeng [Cheng Yi ben]* 紅樓夢 [程乙本]). Beijing: Beijing Tushuguan chubanshe 北京圖書館出版社, 2001, Vol. 2.

Chan Shau Wing (Chen Shourong), ed. *Concise English-Chinese Dictionary*. Stanford, CA: Stanford University Press, 1946.

Charlton, Anne. "Medicinal Uses of Tobacco in History." *Journal of the Royal Society of Medicine* 97.6 (June 2004): 292–296.

Chee, Liz P. Y. *Mao's Bestiary: Medicinal Animals and Modern China*. Durham, NC: Duke University Press, 2021.

Chen Rong 陳榮, et al., ed. *Chinese Medical Literature* (*Zhongyi wenxian* 中醫文獻). Beijing: Zhongyi guji chubanshe 中醫古籍出版社, 2007.

Chinese Dictionary of Medical Books (*Zhongguo yiji da cidian* 中國醫籍大辭典). Ed. the Compilation Committee (*Bianzuan weiyuanhui* 編纂委員會). Shanghai: Shanghai Scientific Press (*Shanghai kexue jishu chubanshe* 上海科學技術出版社), 2002.

A Chinese-English Dictionary (*Han-Ying cidian* 漢英詞典). Beijing: Foreign Language Teaching and Research Press, 2010.

Collection of Rare Books on Asian Medicine, Volume Two (*Tōhō igaku zenhon sōkan, dainisaku* 東方医学善本叢刊，第二冊). Osaka: Oriento shuppansha オリエント出版社, 2001.

Crossley, Pamela Kyle. *Hammer and Anvil: Nomad Rulers at the Forge of the Modern World*. London: Rowman & Littlefield, 2019.

Crow, Sara. "Dew and Flower Essences." *Floracopia*. https://www.floracopeia.com/dew-and-flower-essences. Accessed July 2021.

Chu Ping-Yi (Zhu Pingyi 祝平一). "Qingdai de shazheng: Yige jibing fanchou de dansheng" 清代的痧症：一個疾病範疇的誕生 (Cholera in the Qing Dynasty: The Birth of a Disease Category). *Hanxue yanjiu* 漢學研究 (*Chinese Studies*) 31.3 (September 2014): 193–228.

Daegu Yangnyeongsi Oriental Medicine Museum 大邱藥令市韓醫藥博物館, 2023. http://daegu.go.kr/dgom.

Dashtdar, Mehrab, et al. "The Concept of Wind in Traditional Chinese Medicine." *Journal of Pharmacopuncture* 19.4 (December 2016): 293–302. DOI: 10.3831/KPI.2016.19.030, PMCID: PMC5234349, PMID: 28097039.

De Vries, Ranke. "A Short Tract on Medicinal Uses for Animal Dung." *North American Journal of Celtic Studies* 3.2 (2019): 111–136.

Deng Huichun 鄧慧純. "Have You Had Your Herbs Today?: Welcome to the World of Taiwanese Herbs." *Taiwan Panorama* (April 2023): 76–87.

Dharmananda, Subhuti. "Treatment of Tinnitus, Vertigo, and Meniere's Disease with Chinese Herbs." *Institute for Traditional Medicine*, June 1998. http://www.itmonline.org/arts/tinmen.htm. Accessed July 2020.

Dictionary of Chinese Medical Books (*Zhongguo yiji da cidian* 中國醫籍大辭典). Shanghai: Shanghai kexue jishu chubanshe 上海科學技術出版社, 2002, Vol. 1.

Ditre, Joseph W., et al. "Pain, Nicotine, and Smoking: Research Findings and Mechanistic Considerations." *Psychological Bulletin* 137.6 (November 2011): 1065–1093. DOI: 10.1037/a0025544, PMCID: PMC3202023, NIHMSID: NIHMS324174, PMID: 21967450.

Du, Huan, et al. "Fecal Medicines Used in Traditional Medical System of China: A Systematic Review of Their Names, Original Species, Traditional Uses, and Modern Investigations." *Chinese Medicine* 14.31 (September 2019). DOI: 10.1186/s13020-019-0253-x.

Egbuta, Mary A., Shane McIntosh, Daniel L. E. Waters, Tony Vancov, and Lei Liu. "Biological Importance of Cotton By-Products Relative to Chemical Constituents of the Cotton Plant." *Molecules* 22.1 (January 2017): 93.

Ellis, Andrew, Nigel Wiseman, Ken Boss, and James Cleaver. *Fundamentals of Chinese Acupuncture, Revised Edition.* Taos, NM: Paradigm Publications, 2004.

Essential for Treating Pustules (*Zhiding yaoshu* 治疗要書). Shanghai: Hongda shanshuju 宏大善書局, 1927.

Eyes: A Collection of Medical Prescriptions (*Yanke yaofang huiji* 眼科藥方彙集). In my personal collection, this is a hand-written book of 29 pages hurriedly written by the prescribing doctor with prescriptions for pastes (*gao* 膏) and pills (*wan* 丸) for treating eye afflictions. It has 29 hand-written pages and was purchased in March 2009 in Shandong province, Jinan 山東濟南. 9.5 inch (24.13 cm) h. × 6.75 inch (17.15 cm) w.

Fryklund, Kristin Ingrid, trans. *The Lady of Linshui Pacifies Demons: A Seventeenth-Century Novel.* Seattle: University of Washington Press, 2021. The novel's original title was *Linshui Pingyao* 臨水平妖.

Gao Xiyan 高希言, et al., annot., Xu Jingsheng 許敬生, ed. *Zhenjiu yixue jiaozhu* 針灸易學：校注 (*Acupuncture Made Easy: Proofread*). Zhengzhou, Henan: Henan kexue jishu chubanshe 河南科學技術出版社, 2017.

Goh, S. Y., and K. C. Loh. "Gynaecomastia and the Herbal Tonic Dong Quai." *Singapore Medical Journal* 42.3 (2001): 115–116. PMID: 11405562.

Goodrich, Anne S., *Peking Paper Gods: A Look at Home Worship.* Nettetal: Steyler Verlag, 1991.

Grant, Joanna. *A Chinese Physician: Wang Ji and the Stone Mountain Medical Case Histories.* London: Routledge, 2003.

Greenstone, Gerry. "The History of Bloodletting." *British Columbia Medical Journal* 52.1 (January–February 2010): 12–14.

Guo, Tingwang, Wenfeng Li, Ju Wang, Tiantian Luo, Deshuai Lou, Bochu Wang, and Shilei Hao. "Recombinant Human Hair Keratin Proteins for Halting Bleeding." *Artificial Cells, Nanomedicine, and Biotechnology: An International Journal* 46:sup2 (April 2018): 456–461. DOI: 10.1080/21691401.2018.1459633.

Halimi, Nurfatin Mohdi, Zalifah Mohd Kasim, and Abdul Salam Babji. "Nutritional Composition and Solubility of Edible Bird Nest (Aerodramus fuchiphagus)." *AIP Conference Proceedings,* 1614.476 (February 2014). DOI: 10.1063/1.4895243.

Han, Keguang, et al. "Effects of Lactobacillus Helveticas Fermentation, on the Ca^{2+} Release and Antioxidative Properties of Sheep Bone Hydrolysate." *Korean Journal for Food Science of Animal Resources* 38.6 (December 2018): 1144–1154.

Hinrichs, T. J., and Linda L. Barnes. *Chinese Medicine and Healing: An Illustrated History.* Cambridge, MA: Harvard University Press, 2013.

Hoang Bao Chau, Pho Duc Thuc, et al. *Vietnamese Traditional Medicine.* Hanoi: The Gioi (World) Publishers, 2016.

Hsu Hong-Yen, et al., eds. *Shang Han Lun* (*The Great Classic of Chinese Medicine*). Los Angeles: Oriental Healing Arts Institute, 1981.

Iemoto Sei'ichi 家本誠一. *Outline of Chinese Classical Medicine: The Origins of Herbal Medicine and Acupuncture* (*Chūgoku kodai igaku taikei: Kanpō, shinkyū no genryū* 中国古代医学大系：漢方鍼灸の源流). Tokyo: Seifūsha 靜風社, 2017.

Illness Caused by Heat (*Zhuhuomen* 諸火門). This is a hand-written book of medical prescriptions for illnesses caused by heat (*huo* 火) in my personal collection. Many of the prescriptions are for making pills (*wan* 丸) to treat the illness. Written in the Hall of Middle Harmony (*Zhonghetang* 中和堂) it has 22 folio pages. Purchased in June 2013 in Beijing. 9.5 inch (24.13 cm) h. × 5.75 inch (14.61 cm) w.

Javed, Ahsan, et al. "Turnip (Brassica Rapus): A Natural Health Tono." *Brazilian Journal of Food Technology* 22.5 (January 2019). DOI: 10.1590/1981-6723.25318.

Kendall, Laurel. *Mediums and Magical Things: Statues, Paintings, and Masks in Asian Places*, Oakland, CA: University of California Press, 2022.

Kim, Han, et al. "Cold Hands, Warm Hart." *Lancet Letters* 351.1141 (May 16, 1998): 1492. https://www.thelancet.com/journals/lancet/article/PIIS0140-6736%2805%2978875-9/fulltext. Accessed April 11, 2021.

Kim Jahyun. "Korean Single-Sheet Buddhist Woodblock Illustrated Prints Produced for Protection and Worship." *Religions* 11.12 (2020): 647. DOI: 10.3390/rel11120647.

Kim, Yi-Yung, trans. *The King's Mouthpiece: Institute for the Translation of Korean Classics*. Seoul: Jipmoondang 集文堂, 2019.

Kong, Y. C. (Kong Yun-cheung 江潤祥), trans. and annot. *Huangdi Neijing: A Synopsis with Commentaries* (*Neijing zhiyao yigu* 內經知要譯詁). Hong Kong: The Chinese University Press, 2010.

Kuriyama, Shigehisa. *The Expressiveness of the Body and the Divergence of Greek and Chinese Medicine*. Princeton, NJ: Princeton University Press, 1999.

Kwon, Chan-Young, and Boram Lee. "Acupuncture or Acupressure on *Yintang* (EX HN-3) for Anxiety: A Preliminary Review." *Medical Acupuncture* 30.2 (April 2018): 73–79. DOI: 10.1089/acu2017.1268, PMCID: PMC5908420, PMID: 29682147.

Lee, Jonghyun. "*Hwabyung* and Depressive Symptoms among Korean Immigrants." *Social Work in Mental Health* 13.2 (2015): 159–185. DOI: 10.1080/15332985.2013.812538.

Lee, Ya-Ting. "Principle Study of Head Meridian Acupoint Massage to Stress Release via Grey Data Model Analysis." *Evidence-Based Complementary and Alternative Medicine.* 2016. DOI: 10.1155/2016/4943204. Accessed May 20, 2021.

Leung, Ping Chung. "Use of Animal Fats in Traditional Chinese Medicine." In N. Bhattacharya and P. Stubblefield (eds.), *Regenerative Medicine,* pp. 73–76. London: Springer, 2015.

Levy, Sharon. "Nicotine: It May Have a Good Side." *Harvard Health Publishing.* March 2014. https://www.health.harvard.edu/newsletter_article/Nicotine_It_may_have_a_good_side#:~:text=For%20someone%20who's%20agitated%2C%20nicotine,manner%20as%. Accessed August 10, 2020.

Lim, Hyun Hwa, et al. "Anti-Inflammatory and Antiobesity Effects of Mulberry Leaf and Fruit Extract on High Fat Diet-Induced Obesity." *National Library of Medicine* 238.10 (October 2013): 1160–1169. DOI: 10.1177/1535370213498982.

Ling, Yang, Dan Yang, and Wenlong Shao. "Understanding Vomiting from the Perspective of Traditional Chinese Medicine." *Annals of Palliative Medicine*1.2 (July 2012): 143–160. DOI: 10.3978/j.issn.2224-5820.2012.07.03. http://apm.amegroups.com/article/view/1040/1267. Accessed May 21, 2021.

Lingying yaowang zhenjing 靈應藥王真經 (*True Classic of the Lingying Medicine King*). Shiyan, Hubei: Saiwudang Daoists Association of Taishan Monastery, 2014.

Liu 劉氏. *Headaches* (*Toutong* 頭痛 / *touteng* 頭疼). Shandong, Jiaozhou-fu, late Qing.

Liu Bangming 劉幫明. *Inspection of Face and Body for Diagnosis of Diseases,* 2nd ed. Beijing: Foreign Languages Press, 2006.

Liu, Fei, et al. "Antitumor Effect and Mechanism of Gecko on Human Esophageal Carcinoma Cell Lines in Vitro and Xenografted Sarcoma 180 in Kunming Mice." *World Journal of Gastroenterology* 14.25 (July 2008): 3990–3996. DOI: 10.3748/wjg.14.3990.

Liu Lihong. *Classical Chinese Medicine.* Ed. Heiner Fruehauf. Trans. Gabriel Weiss, Henry Buchtel, and Sabine Wilms. Hong Kong: The Chinese University Press, 2019.

Liu, Yan. *Healing with Poisons: Potent Medicines in Medieval China.* Seattle, WA: Washington University Press, 2021.

Lo, Vivienne, et al. *Imagining Chinese Medicine.* Leiden: Brill, 2018.

Lo, Y. L., and S. L. Cui. "Acupuncture and the Modulation of Cortical Excitability." *NeuroReport* 14.9 (July 2003): 1229–1231.

Maciocia, Giovanni 馬萬里. "Phlegm-Heat in Chinese Medicine." https://giovanni-maciocia.com/phlegm-hea/. Accessed June 2021.

Mair, Victor. "The Biography of Hua-t'o from the 'History of the Three Kingdoms.'" In Victor H. Mair (ed.), *The Columbia Anthology of Traditional Chinese Literature*, pp. 688–696. New York: Columbia University Press, 1994.

Matthews' Chinese-English Dictionary. Originally published in 1931. Revised American Edition published in Taiwan, 1974.

Mayanagi Makoto 直柳誠. *Research on the Yellow Emperor's Medical Texts* (*Kōtei iseki kenkyū* 黃帝医籍研究). Tokyo: Kyūko shoin 汲古書院, 2014.

Menzies, Nicholas K. *Ordering the Myriad Things: From Traditional Knowledge to Scientific Botany in China.* Seattle: University of Washington Press, 2021.

Mitchell, Damo, and Spencer Hill. *The Yellow Monkey Emperor's Classic of Chinese Medicine.* London: Singing Dragon, 2016.

Nayak, R., et al. "Asterixis (flapping tremors) as an Outcome of Complex Psychotropic Drug Interaction." *Journal of Neuropsychiatry and Clinical Neuroscience* 24.1 (Winter 2012): 27–29.

New Age Chinese-English Dictionary (*Xinshidai Han-Ying da cidian* 新時代漢英大詞典). Beijing: The Commercial Press, 2007.

Otsuka Keisetsu 大塚敬節, et al. *Kanpō dai'iten* 漢方大医典 (Dictionary of Chinese Medicine). Tokyo: Tōto shobō 東都書房, 1957.

Pannu, A. K., and S. Pannu. "Scrofula." *QJM: An International Journal of Medicine* 110.8 (August 2017): 535. DOI: 10.1093/qjmed/hcx098. Accessed June 2021.

Panthati, Murali Krishna, K. N. V. Rao, S. Sandhya, and David Banjii. "A Review on Phytochemical, Ethnomedical and Pharmacological Studies on Genus *Sophora*, Fabaceae." *Revista Brasileira de Farmacognosia* 22.5 (September–October 2012): 1145–1154.

Park, Enkyo, et al. "Anti-Inflammatory Activity of Mulberry Leaf Extract Through Inhibition of NF-κB." *Journal of Functional Foods* 5.1 (January 2013): 178–186.

Pathirana, W., et al. "Transcranial Route of Brain Targeted Delivery of Methadone in Oil." *Indian Journal of Pharmaceutical Science* 71.3 (May–June 2009): 264–269.

Precious Imperial Compendium of the Medical Profession, Vol. 3: Correct Procedures in External Medicine for the Heart-Mind (*Yuzuan yicong jinjian, juan san: Bianji waike xinfa yaojue* 御纂醫宗金鑒，卷三：編輯外科心法要訣).

Precious Imperial Compendium of the Medical Profession, Vol. 17: Revised Annotations on Cold Injuries (*Yuzuan yicong jinjian, juan shiqi: Dingzheng Shanghanlun zhu zhengwu pian* 御纂醫宗金鑒，卷十七：訂正傷寒論註正誤篇). 1793.

Return to Health Pill (*Huitian zaizao wan* 回天再造丸). This is a book of medical prescriptions (*yaopu* 藥譜) with prescriptions for making pills. It has 59 pages of hand-written medical recipes. In my personal collection. Bought it in Shenyang 瀋陽 in June 2011. On handmade paper and covered in accountant's blue gauze, its dates could be anywhere from the late 1800s to the late 1920s. 9.5 inch (24.13 cm) h. × 10 inch (25.4 cm) w.

Rogaski, Ruth. *Knowing Manchuria: Environments, the Senses, and Natural Knowledge on an Asian Borderland.* Chicago: University of Chicago Press, 2022.

Rouse, Jillian G., and Mark E. Van Dyke. "A Review of Keratin-Based Biomaterials for Biomedical Applications." *Materials (Basel)* 3.2 (February 2010): 999–1014. DOI: 10.3390/ma3020999, PMCID: PMC5513517.

Sanchez-Ramosa, Juan R. "The Rise and Fall of Tobacco as a Botanical Medicine." *Journal of Herbal Medicine* 22 (August 2020). DOI: 10.1016/j.hermed.2020.100374.

Schell, Jonathan, trans. *Discussion of Cold Damage with Annotations.* Portland, OR: Chinese Medicine Database, 2018.

Schonebaum, Andrew. *Novel Medicine: Healing, Literature, and Popular Knowledge in Early Modern China.* Seattle: University of Washington Press, 2016.

Seabrooks, Lauren, and Longqin Hua. "Insects: An Underrepresented Resource for the Discovery of Biologically Active Natural Products." *Acta Pharmaceutica Sinica B* 7.4 (July 2017): 409–426. DOI: 10.1016/j.apsb.2017.05.001.

Shen, Yoshi F., et al. "Randomized Clinical Trial of Acupuncture for Myofascial Pain of the Jaw Muscles." *Journal of Orofacial Pain* 23.4 (Fall 2009): 353–359. PMCID: PMC2894813, NIHMSID: NIHMS209743, PMID: 19888488.

Shen, Yu. "Earthworms in Traditional Chinese Medicine." In *Advances of the 4th International Oligochaeta Taxonomy Meeting, Zoology in the Middle East, Supplementum 2*, pp. 171–173. Heidelberg: Kasparek Verlag, 2010.

Shimbara, Hisashi, et al. "Effects of Manual Acupuncture with Sparrow Pecking on Muscle Blood Flow of Normal and Denervated Hindlimb in Rats." *Acupuncture in Medicine* 26.3 (October 2008): 149–159. DOI: 10.1136/aim.26.3.149.

Sierwald, Petra, et al. "Current Status of the Myriapod Class Diplopoda (Millipedes): Taxonomic Diversity and Phylogeny." *Annual Review of Entomology* 52.1 (2007): 401–420. DOI: 10.1146/annurev.ento.52.111805.090210, PMID: 17163800.

Silberstein, Rachel. *A Fashionable Century: Textile Artistry and Commerce in the Late Qing.* Seattle, WA: University of Washington Press, 2020.

Strickmann, Michel, and Barnard Faure, eds. *Chinese Magical Medicine.* Stanford, CA; Stanford University Press, 2002.

Suleski, Ronald. *Daily Life for the Common People of China, 1850 to 1950: Understanding Chaoben Culture.* Leiden: Brill, 2018.

Unschuld, Paul U. *Traditional Chinese Medicine: Heritage and Adaptation.* Trans. Birdie Andrews. New York: Columbia University Press, 2018.

Veith, Ilza, trans. *The Yellow Emperor's Classic of Internal Medicine.* Berkeley, CA: University of California Press, 2002.

Wallnofer, Heinrich, and Anna Von Rottauscher. *Chinese Folk Medicine.* Trans. Marion Palmedo. New York: Bell Publishing, 1965.

Wang Bin 王彬 and Xu Xiushan 徐秀珊, eds. *Dictionary of Beijing Place Names (Beijing Diming Dian* 北京地名典*).* Revised Edition. Beijing: Zhongguo wenlian chubanshe 中國文聯出版社, 2008.

Wang Xiaoying 王曉鷹 and Zhang Yihua 章宜華, eds. *English-Chinese Chinese-English Medical Dictionary (Yinghan hanying yixue cidian* 英漢漢英醫學詞典*).* Beijing: Foreign Language Teaching and Research Press 外語教學與研究出版社, 2008.

Wiseman, Nigel, and Andrew Ellis. *Fundamentals of Chinese Medicine, Revised Edition.* Brookline, MA, 1995.

Wu, Feifei. "Deer Antler Base as a Traditional Chinese Medicine: A Review of its Traditional Uses, Chemistry and Pharmacology." *Journal of Ethnopharmacology* 145.2 (January 30, 2013): 403–415.

Wu Peijin 吳佩瑾 and Liu Weizhi 劉威志. "'Yingxiang yu yiliao de lishi' zhuti jihua: Zhuanfang Li Zhende, Zhu Pingyi jiaoshou"「影像與醫療的歷史」主題計劃：專訪李貞德、祝平一教授 ("The History of Medical Healing and Illustrations" Thematic Project: Interviews with Professors Li Zhende and Chu Pingyi). *Ming-Qing yanjiu tongxun* 明清研究通訊 (Ming-Qing Research Bulletin) 19 (May 2011). http://mingching.sinica.edu.tw/Academic_Detail/149.

Wu, Yi-Li. *The Injured Body: A Social History of Medicine for Wounds in Late Imperial China.* Forthcoming.

Xing, G. S., et al. "Treating 19 Cases of Epilepsy with a Combination of Acupuncture and Herbs." *Journal of Acupuncture Clinical Application* 15.3 (1999): 13–14.

Xu, Fabao, and Chenjin Jin. "Acupuncture and Ocular Penetration." *Ophthalmology* 128.2 (February 2021): 217. DOI: 10.1016/j.ophtha.2020.09.024.

Yan Shiyi 嚴世藝, ed. *Zhongguo yiji tongkao* 中國醫籍通考 (*Chinese Medical Books*). Shanghai: Shanghai zhongyixueyuan chubanshe 上海中醫學院出版社, 1990.

Yang, Fan, et al. "Thermostable Potassium Channel-Inhibiting Neurotoxins in Processed Scorpion Medicinal Material Revealed by Proteomic Analysis: Implications of Its Pharmaceutical Basis in Traditional Chinese Medicine." *Journal of Proteomics* (July 2019). PMID: 31279926, DOI: 10.1016/j.jprot.2019.103435.

Yang Huasen 楊華森, et al., eds. *Jianming Zhongyi zidian* 簡明中醫字典 (*Basic Chinese Medical Dictionary*). Guiyang: Guizhou renmin chubanshe 貴州人民出版社, 1985.

Yang Zhenhai 楊真海. *The Yellow Emperor's Inner Transmission of Acupuncture* (*Huangdi neizhen* 黃帝內針). Ed. Liu Lihong. Trans. Sabine Wilms. Intro. Heiner Fruehauf. Hong Kong: The Chinese University of Hong Kong Press, 2020.

Yingyong quanji 應用全集 (*Useful Collection*). This is a hand-written book of 87 pages in my personal collection. It contains petitions to the deities asking to be cured of illness. The *wuchen* 戊辰 year is referenced, which could be 1868 or 1928. The text has many references to the Great Qing Dynasty (*Daqing* 大清), and yet this appears to be made of machine-made paper with printed columns of a type common in the Republic, so either date could be correct. Purchased in Beijing in March 2009. 7.12 inch (18.08 cm) h. × 3.5 inch (8.89 cm) w.

Yu, Lin. "Wang Shixiong's Medicine Career." *Chinese Medicine and Culture* 3.4 (2020): 254–256. https://www.cmaconweb.org/article.asp?issn=2589-9627; year=2020;volume=3;issue=4;spage=254;epage=256;aulast=Yu.

Zhang Zhibin, and Paul U. Unschuld, eds. *Dictionary of the Ben Cao Gang Mu, Vol. I: Chinese Historical Illness Terminology.* University of California Press, 2015.

Zhuang Huafeng 莊華峰 and Fang Baiying 方百盈, eds. *Dictionary of Chinese Traditional Health* (*Zhongguo chuantong yangshengxue cidian* 中國傳統養生學辭典). Nanning: Guangxi jiaoyu chubanshe 廣西教育出版社, 1996.

INDEX